Whole

Navigating the Trauma of Pregnancy Loss

Heather Dolson, R.N.

Heather on Health

Contents

One

Introduction

♥

First, I am deeply sorry that you had to pick this book, whether it's because of your pregnancy loss or because you want to make sense of a loved one's pain in this heartbreaking moment.

Life is a strange paradox. Like a coin, it has two sides. The beautiful moments will be great and wholesome. It's like a treasure chest of fine, rare, and invaluable jewels. In the good moments, life will show you its stunning colors, but as they say, "*the stream would have no song if it wouldn't have rocks in its beds.*" This means we must also experience the darker shades, the sad moments. In the dark moments, we'll understand the depth of life. We love, and we lose; no one can explain it. It's just the way it is. You can't have one without the other. You will inevitably confront grief if you open yourself to love. You may try to avoid grief, but then you will never experience love, one of the most precious gifts of life. In the end, therefore, it's evident that love and loss are part of what makes us fully alive.

Of all the losses we'll experience in life, pregnancy loss is one of the most traumatic. Because pregnancy is bundled up with heightened emotions, vulnerability, expectations, and hope for the future, its loss can feel like the tragic end of a promising journey or the loss of a beautiful dream. As it is, pregnancy changes our identity, role, and physical status, all of which spark strong emotions. You get attached quickly, especially when the details start to trickle in; the gender, due date, sex, and physical growth. Even amid uncertainty and physical and emotional discomfort, there is hope, a powerful connection to the growing baby, and the expectation of a possible relationship with someone you've never met before.

Pregnancy sets us on a journey of physical, emotional, and hormonal changes, whose momentum can sometimes be compelling. The effects of pregnancy on us are complicated and profound. Because a lot of intimacy and vulnerability is involved, whichever way the pregnancy came to be, part of us is shattered when it is lost. You may feel like life has lost direction, the train of life has gone off the rails, and the resulting darker shades of life that come in fear, pain, and heartbreak have taken over. Your reaction to pregnancy loss is fitting, as upsetting as it may be. Mourning the loss of someone or something so meaningful and deserving of our love, care, and attention is not an easy thing. The pain of pregnancy loss is only familiar to those who've experienced it. It changes you forever; there is nothing like getting over it; nothing normal to go back to.

Indeed, studies show that pregnancy loss is common. Approximately 10-20% of pregnancies will be miscarried, medically defined as the loss of pregnancy within the first 20 weeks of gestation. Furthermore, 1% of recognized pregnancies will end up in stillbirth, which is the loss of a pregnancy after the 20th week. However, your life is yours alone; no one can live your pain for you. People can help you through it, but the depths of pain and sadness, however deep they go, are yours to feel.

It's therefore heartbreaking when some people act like *"you are overreacting,"* or *"making it bigger than it* is," or "*it's just the loss of a potential baby*." Pregnancy loss is devastating because it's the loss of a future, the loss of a generation. The loss of a lifetime of beautiful memories that would have been. You are only left with the "ifs" and "maybes." They don't understand; no one can. Some people will say that you should be glad you weren't too attached and that you should be happy it never happened sooner. But you fell in love when the second line appeared on the test. You knew you wanted them to be here.

Pregnancy loss is a painful, traumatic, tragic, terrible, life-altering experience, so, NO! You are not overreacting. You know what you lost:

You'll never see your baby's first steps, smile, or teeth.

You'll never get the chance to comfort them when they cry.

You'll never see them running up to you or get to pick them up.

There'll never be the first day of preschool, kindergarten, high school, or college; not for this baby.

There will never be a first dance, graduation, or a wedding.

No first drives, first dates, or watching them become parents to their kids or grandparents.

When you grieve, it's not about the attachment or lack of it because of how long you were pregnant, as many assume; your heart breaks for the future, all the hopes, dreams, and memories that will never see the light of day. You are holding this book right now, so I know you are mourning the possibilities and the future that will never be. My experience as a registered nurse with a passion for mental health, death and dying, loss, and the human experience on earth mean that I customarily see what desperation feels like. I know how separation can make you pick up every book, blog, or article about loss and grief in the hope that it will relieve the pain.

I want to tell you from the beginning that I hope this book will be helpful, but it won't rescue you from the pain of loss and grief. I wish I were in that place to take away the pain, but nothing in this world will provide you with that. No book written under the sun will help you escape your grief. There is no shortcut through grief, no fast cut through pain and loss. You have to live it and feel it. This book isn't a lifeboat sent to save you from drowning. Sadly, we had to meet under these circumstances, but in this book, I am offering you the gift of friendship in this challenging time, a life preserver that will make you feel less lonely as you navigate the bumpy road ahead.

In all my years working as a registered nurse and life coach, I have met many women, couples, and families dealing with unbearable and unimaginable loss and grief. People that have mental health problems come from all walks of life;

some people struggle with substance abuse that has led to addictions, endless cycles of homelessness, prostitution, and self-harm. Others are dealing with generational patterns of abuse, grief, and trauma caused by violence. My experiences with mental health have empowered me in different ways and made me an advocate for people who've been dealt unimaginable horror and difficulties. I have, for many years, personally studied and practiced yoga, meditation, and always had a keen fascination in human psychology and personal development. I do believe that challenges are put in our path to help us evolve as human beings. I care deeply for people going through loss, grief, and pain. I know this is important, valuable work.

I have also learned that those who've suffered loss and grief have wisdom that can benefit the world. As it is, modern society's version of dealing with grief is wholly broken. Our culture is afraid to feel and treats grief as a messy, scary emotion that we should deal with quickly and get over as soon as possible. For this reason, many still harbor outdated beliefs about grief, giving it a face and timeline. They have assumptions about how grief should look and how long it should last. We must open ourselves to the depths of real human existence, where loss and grief are inevitable. We'll appreciate life and feelings if we open ourselves to human experiences.

We will only stop judging, correcting, and shaming people in their grief.

Many people who've lost a pregnancy admit that they've been encouraged to "put the past behind them," "get over it," and stop talking about the baby who is no longer with them. Some people will admonish you and advise you to move on because "these deaths teach you to appreciate life." Sometimes, even those with pure intentions will end up hurting you. Even when told with good intentions, endless clichés and unsolicited advice may seem insensitive and dismissive. You may feel alone, judged, misunderstood. It may not even be that people around you are dismissive or insensitive; some may not know how to help because they've never known the pain of losing a pregnancy. It is sad because, in this situation, no one wins; you feel misunderstood, and your loved ones feel helpless and ignorant of your grief.

In the end, how we experience love and extend our friendship to those who grieve is the true test of the bond of love we have for each other. It is in listening without judgment or being pushy. It is about helping each other and pulling them up when they are drowning in grief and sadness. It's about thinking; what would this person need? What do they feel, and how can I be of help? The answers to these questions are critical, and I hope this book will deliver those answers. Although being a nurse has coloured my background and I know you may be looking for medical-related answers to pregnancy loss; I also know that amid grief, the last thing anyone wants is to be blindsided by a clinical book full of medical jargon that will leave them feeling cold and scared.

What you need is daily support, a friend, if you want to call it that, who can walk with you through the grief and give you hope. You are walking in a dark place, a black hole that lacks understanding and is empty of grace and love. That's why I am switching a light on so that in this book, you'll find light in the midst of that horrid, grief-filled space.

This book borrows a lot from my education and experience as a registered nurse, my personal experience as a single mother who has dealt with loss and grief, a holistic life coach who guides women to make space for the shadows and release shame and guilt, and a woman with a renewed connection to my womb who has healed sexual trauma and had the experience of bonding to my unborn child in the womb. It is informed by my extensive research in mental health following death, dying, loss, and the human experience on earth. I would describe it as an extension of my clinical work with people who've lived the days, months, and years following loss and tragedy.

I know that everyone deals with and describes grief differently, which is why this book isn't just about my opinions. I have included other people's views, so you can see things from different angles. I am also aware that the experiences of pregnancy loss vary widely based on biological, cultural, and socioeconomic factors that are never constant. For this reason, I will say that this book doesn't claim to have all the answers, nor is it a representation of all the experiences that people who've lost pregnancies have and will go through. You are the expert in your grief and loss, so I suggest you treat this book as a guide. This book doesn't replace medical intervention available to you through therapy, advice, or help.

This book is written for everyone who feels overwhelmed after the tragedy and loss of a baby. It is for you if you want to find peace and wholeness in the midst of grief. Traumatic experiences can be an opportunity to learn and grow, transmute the pain, and experience personal evolution and transformation. It's for all women and men looking for tactical advice on navigating relationships with partners, family, friends, and with themselves during this loss and in the aftermath. If you wonder if you'll ever feel whole again or if whatever you feel is normal, this book is for you. It teaches you how to reframe your relationship with grief so you can give yourself the empathy, understanding, and compassion you so freely give to others.

I'll be glad if this book helps you, even in a small way. I will be ecstatic if it will make you feel less alone.

Two

Acknowledge the Loss

♥

It's heartbreaking to hear that one in every four pregnancies will be lost to miscarriage. Another 2.6 million babies are stillborn, with more than half dying during birth. As high as these numbers are, there is still speculation that these may be low-ball figures. After all, lost pregnancies are harder to track. If pregnancy loss is as common as it sounds, why is our society still closed-minded about something acknowledged by so many? Why is pregnancy loss still a taboo subject and a stigmatized experience? Pregnancy loss is a subject that is distressfully under-studied and under-resourced. There is a widespread lack of understanding about this sensitive yet significant subject.

Every person deals with grief differently, and pregnancy loss varies widely. Still, even statistics from the World Health Organization show that the stigma and shame associated with pregnancy loss cut across all cultures worldwide. One common example of miscarriage-related stigma is the "first-trimester rule." Many women decide not to tell others they are pregnant until the 13th to 16th week of pregnancy. Why? Because the risk of loss is greater during the early weeks of pregnancy. For this reason, many will decide to keep quiet. If you followed this "rule" only to lose the pregnancy within the first trimester, your loved ones are only just learning that you were even pregnant. Then they have to learn about the loss as well.

Because many women don't feel comfortable sharing their pregnancy early, they choose silence if they lose the pregnancy. They'd instead isolate themselves and deal with the pain alone. Therefore, the secrecy associated with the pregnancy extends to the loss, which only increases the stigma surrounding pregnancy loss. The stigma and shame associated with pregnancy loss may lead to isolation and disconnection from loved ones. Ultimately, many women and couples feel trapped and alone in their grief. Most feel like no one gets it, and no one knows how to help.

This level of compounded grief is unimaginable and disturbing.

Pregnancy loss *is* loss, and it is an *actual* loss, regardless of how and when the baby is lost. Every woman deserves validation and acknowledgment after losing a pregnancy, at a few weeks or months. Every person who experiences this kind of loss deserves respect, dignified attention, and emotional, psychological, and physical support. A recent study on women who miscarried reported that many wished they had told their loved ones the news early on in their pregnancy so they didn't have to grieve in silence following a miscarriage in the first trimester.

Many parents choose to grieve in silence, and that's okay because there isn't a right or wrong way to grieve. But if there is one thing we must acknowledge, it should be that a loss is a loss, and grief is grief. Everything you are feeling is normal, and you are allowed to mourn your child. Your body was holding a life once, and then suddenly, it wasn't. It shouldn't matter how brief or prolonged that moment was.

Seeing that there wasn't a body to grieve or a funeral, many people assume that the loss may not be equal to someone who was already with you. This is entirely untrue. Why should mourning be related to the length of time you were pregnant? Sadly, the grief of women who miscarried early is even less socially acceptable than the pain of someone who miscarried later. It's a common myth that a pregnancy lost earlier is less painful, and the woman feels less grief.

We are completely blind to the realities of having a miscarriage. You'd be surprised by the number of people who take it lightly. In fact, people who've never been through a miscarriage or medical termination of a pregnancy admit that they don't understand the emotions associated with pregnancy loss. Isn't it like the monthly period, a more challenging one, maybe? No, it is not. Miscarriage and crampy heavy periods are two different things. A miscarriage or medical termination is like the death of a child following intense labor and birth. We can even say it is worse, more challenging, and more painful than birth. You experience the same amount of physical pain and labor associated with birth and the emotional attachment to a baby that you'll never hold or breastfeed. Instead, you are only left with a deep sense of emptiness following the pregnancy loss.

The identity fracture associated with pregnancy loss is something we must acknowledge if we are to understand why mourning all pregnancies is okay. Many studies show that as soon as they realize they are pregnant, many expectant parents adopt their mom/dad identities. This means that as soon as you know you are pregnant, your identity starts to change, and in your mind, you start seeing yourself as a mother or a father – or a father or mother to be.

There is a good chance some names have been picked already, you've thought of their eye and hair color, what they'll look like, what they'll study and what kind of person they'll be. If this is true, would it not make sense for someone to mourn a baby who's just a few weeks old? Regardless of how early or far you are in your pregnancy, a miscarriage is a brutal, heartbreaking message that there is no longer that possibility; a chance at being a parent no longer exists, at least not now and not with this child. You have every right to grieve this possibility ending and this baby, no matter how short the pregnancy was.

It would have been better if pregnancy loss didn't negate that identity, the possibility of parenthood. But as it is, society doesn't have the "right" language for parents who've lost their children through miscarriages or medical termination. What's the proper term for a parent whose child isn't physically present after pregnancy loss, especially if they don't have other kids? The lack of legitimate language within our culture and the stigma surrounding this sensitive topic fuel the difficulties associated with life after losing a child. In recent years, terms like "angel babies" have emerged and are now associated with babies lost differently. These terms are important because they help open up the space for these difficult conversations. If people can have these conversations, the stigma associated with pregnancy loss could be reduced.

Disenfranchised grief

It's in our nature to mourn when we lose something. But what if your grief is tinged by guilt?

People tend to recognize the loss of a spouse or a family member as a significant loss. For example, when someone you know learns that you lost a parent, they'll send a card, show up with food and come to comfort you. But would they do the same when you lose your pet, your mobility, a client, or fail an important test? What if you just lost a pregnancy? Would people react the same way? A few would, but there is a chance most people will ignore or dismiss the loss.

If this happens, you may wonder, "*am I overreacting*?" "*Maybe I am too sad*?" And someone might have said it to you already, *"it's not like it was a child."* Maybe that negative voice inside your head has been whispering that you shouldn't mourn the loss of a miscarriage or medical termination when you already have other kids or because you can still have other children. But why should the type of loss matter if you genuinely cared and were emotionally and physically invested in something.

All grief is valid, no matter the type of loss.

Sadly, society doesn't recognize all grief as grief. For this reason, many people deal with their sorrow silently because they feel they aren't entitled to it or that no one understands. If your grief isn't acknowledged, the healing process becomes difficult. We must admit that Kenneth Doka, who coined the term "disenfranchised grief" in 1989, was well ahead of his time. He accurately described the society we live in today. As a bereavement expert, he recognized that loss doesn't just happen when people die.

Disenfranchised grief is the invalidated hidden sorrow that most people are forced to endure because society minimizes or misunderstands their loss. By failing to recognize certain types of loss, people make it harder for others to express their sadness or start the healing process.

The bereavement expert, Kenneth Doka, admits that it's imperative to mourn every kind of loss, whether or not it is recognized by society. It's important to grieve when you feel like you've lost something. Grief is a normal reaction to loss. Why do people interpret loss as death only? Don't dismiss your feelings to align with societal expectations. Recognizing the loss is the first step toward healing. Unless you find ways to deal with and address them, your feelings of loss will never go away.

> "We say depression and anxiety are conditions of the mind, while grief is a condition of the heart. The grief associated with loss must be dealt with on the emotional and heart level. You can't think your way into better grief." ~ David Defoe

Grief stays with us, especially when we don't take enough time to process the pain and grieve appropriately. When you bottle things inside, they'll slowly build up and overwhelm you. You'll get angry, bitter, and apathetic. You'll realize that you have some internal issues you need to address. Over time, you become an irritable person, someone who's easily triggered. No one wants to be around an irritable person or someone who projects their issues onto others.

Deal with your loss now. Talk to someone now. Tell them how you feel, and allow them to support you during your time of mourning. Tell them how they can help you during this trying time. If you don't feel comfortable talking to family or friends, find a professional. This is what therapists do; they help you deal with and process grief. If you can find a community, that would be very helpful. Support is critical in times of sorrow. Being around understanding people can be powerful. The most harmful thing you can do while grieving is isolating yourself.

Because society doesn't recognize disenfranchised grief as grief, it hasn't created room for rituals designed to mourn these losses. Maybe there is no body, a casket, or burial, which means you'll never get closure. You are in this alone and must learn to navigate independently with nothing close to an end in sight. This loss is yours; you don't have to wait for people to acknowledge it. Design your conclusionary ritual, one that makes sense to you. Write in a journal, plant a flower or a tree in their memory, get a tattoo if you are a fan of that, or create beautiful art that will act as a reminder. Grief is an intimate thing. It's very personal, so you are the only one who knows how best to process it and the befitting ritual.

"We don't get over losses. We must figure out a way to move beyond them." ~ David Defoe

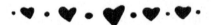

The 5 Stages of Grief

Grief has no formula, no right or wrong way to do it. As I have said throughout this text, everyone deals with it uniquely. However, many people admit they felt overwhelmed and confused after a loss. This is a natural process; others may argue that it is a necessary part of healing. Healing is a complicated process that takes time and requires patience and understanding.

Research has been done on this very sensitive issue, with many experts dedicating their time to studying the emotions associated with grief. Elisabeth Kubler-Ross is one such expert, highly respected in the medical community; she studied human emotions following a loss for many years and came up with a theory – The Five Stages of Grief and Loss, highlighted by the Kubler-Ross Model. She concluded that people go through five primary emotions when mourning; denial, anger, bargaining, depression, and acceptance.

Over the last few decades, these five stages of grief have evolved massively. Indeed, many people misunderstood them, making them a little controversial. But as you read about these five stages of grief, it's important to understand that the goal has never been about tucking these wild emotions into perfect bundles. They are responses that many people will experience, but there is no standard response or expectation on how anyone should react to grief. The five stages of grief are nothing more than a framework, a set of tools that help us understand our emotions and learn to live after loss. They are not a timeline or "traffic stops" that everyone will go through in the exact order or must even go through. I hope the knowledge you learn from these stages will prepare you for all grief-related emotions. In this section, I will discuss the first three stages of grief.

Shock

This will be the first stage for some people following the sad news. The news sounds like a massive blow, and you may be trying to make sense of it, but you cannot. This first stage can last for a few hours or several days. For other people, shock may reappear throughout the grieving process. A new wave of shock may reappear after a trigger or painful memory.

Shock may look like this:

- An inability to or difficulty expressing your emotions.

- You may have trouble understanding the impact of the news or its meaning. For example, following pregnancy loss, you may have difficulty deciding on the treatment options.

- Numbness or paralysis

- You may be overwhelmed with emotions.

- You may feel weary and in need of a break.

Anger

Pain can sometimes manifest as anger. The intense anger you feel might surprise you or your loved ones, but it's not an abnormal reaction to grief. Anger following loss has a purpose. You know the other person isn't to blame, but you'll still be angry at them for leaving or causing you so much pain. You may also feel angry at strangers, loved ones, your partner, God, Source, or inanimate objects, including life itself. You may ask yourself, "why did it have to be me?" "Why me?" "What did I do to deserve something as painful as this?"

But anger is, should I say, a good thing? When you get the sad news of a loss, you may feel numb and disconnected from the world. Anger, on the contrary, is an emotion, a feeling. Even if you feel angry, at least you feel something. Many cultures despise anger and look at it as a destructive emotion, so you may feel guilty for feeling this way. You must remember, however, that there is pain beneath the anger, and it's a step towards healing. You may also feel other emotions, including rage, bitterness, irritability, and anxiety, which are part of the healing process.

Bargaining

You can also call this stage "false hope." Bargaining is synonymous with wishful thinking. You may think about everything you are willing to sacrifice if your life could return to the way it used to be. You'll find yourself creating "what if" and "if only scenarios" in your head and wishing you could have done things differently. Bargaining is usually accompanied by regret and guilt. You are, in your mind, trying to take control of the situation and restore things to how they were. It's hard, but bargaining isn't uncommon, and it helps you heal and move on from the painful experience.

Why you shouldn't say certain things

We will all run into or come to know someone who has lost a pregnancy at some point in our lives. In trying to be empathetic and caring, many people end up saying things that make the grieving person feel worse. Avoid phrases that come across as dismissive, judgmental, accusatory or anything that downplays or minimizes the grieving person's loss.

Avoid any of the following phrases or anything close to or resembling them:

"*Don't worry; you'll get over it before you know it*"

Many women struggle with pregnancy loss for years. Some never get over it completely. They learn to accept it, but it's always a painful reminder of what could have been. It will always be a sad loss. Instead, say something more supportive like, "*I'm here to listen if you need to talk.*" As they struggle with their new reality, grieving people would rather have someone who can comfort, listen and understand without telling them how they are supposed to feel.

"*You can always try again*."

Well-meaning people commonly say this phrase, but it takes away from the person's pain. What if they feel like they don't want to try again? It's okay that you are trying to cheer them up and have them move on, but they are probably not ready to hear this or haven't decided whether they want to try again. When you say this, you sound pushy and dismissive of their current loss. Even if they try, that child will never replace the one they've just lost. Instead, you can say something like, "*it's okay if you need time to process this loss*."

"*You're lucky; you weren't that far into the pregnancy*," or "*it's okay, you didn't know them yet*."

A loss is a loss, whether a few weeks or eight months old.

It may sound like minimizing the loss will be helpful, but I promise you it's not. It will only serve to exacerbate their sense of loss, and they'll see that you are trying to minimize it. Just show the grieving person that you will be there, helping them through it all if they need anything. Show them empathy instead, "*This is painful, and I am very sorry*." Acknowledge the pain they have and offer support where they need it.

"Maybe this child wasn't meant to be" or **_"it was for the best."_**

Just listen. How do you know what was meant to be and what wasn't? Best for whom? And even if it's true that it wasn't meant to be or was for the best, saying it doesn't help. I know you want to make your loved one in emotional pain feel better, and this could mean saying things that you think will make them _"get over their loss sooner."_ Resist the urge to try to cheer them up. Friendship isn't always about staying positive. Sometimes it's about holding space and sitting with them in their pain and being with them through it.

"Miscarriage is common. Many women miscarry but have healthy babies later."

You are minimizing the current loss. This phrase doesn't give the women enough space to grieve without being judged. Maybe she is still scared of what could happen if she tries again or has decided she won't try again so that this comment will be misplaced. Maybe the doctor told her some difficult news, saying this would only look like you are adding salt to the injury.

"This is nature's way of taking care of genetic abnormalities. The child would have suffered, you know?"

As well-meaning as this phrase may sound, it doesn't provide the grieving parent any comfort. It just breaks their heart more. They probably loved the baby already, genetic abnormalities or not. Some miscarriages indeed happen due to medical complications, but you don't know this for a fact. Sometimes miscarriages just happen. Phrases like these minimize the loss and belittle what might have been the happiest moment of their lives. You can instead say, "I *am sorry for your pain. My thoughts are with you in this difficult moment.*"

"Is there a chance you did something you weren't supposed to?"

This is the most insensitive thing you can say to someone who just lost a pregnancy. It comes off as accusatory and judgmental. It's okay to wonder why it happened, but asking it this way implies blame and may make the woman feel guilty even when they did nothing wrong. Besides, you only make them feel bad for something they probably had no control over. Saying this only adds to their destructive guilt. Saying something along the lines, "*you'll need to take good care of your physical and mental health. I am here to help with whatever you need, a hug, dinner, listening, etc.*"

"It happened for a reason."

Pregnancy loss is hard to process, just like any other loss. Everything you say needs to reflect this. You have very good intentions when you say this, but it doesn't help because the parents don't see that reason right now. This response invalidates and minimizes their grief following the loss of their baby. You end up losing the bigger picture by trying to make sense of the loss and putting it into perspective. It could be that the parents already imagined and planned their lives with the baby in it.

"*You'll be okay in no time.*"

While this comment may sound innocent, it's unnecessary. Every one of us processes grief differently. There isn't a set time to process this kind of loss. Even the parents may process this loss differently, so you are in no place to say how soon or how long their grieving process should take. You don't know if they'll be okay soon, so saying this only serves to invalidate their experience. It also gives them an expectation of how long it should take them to get over it, which can be unrealistic.

"*You have other kids, so be grateful for them….*"

Yes, they have other kids, but they wanted this baby too. You'll come across as insensitive and dismissive in this situation, so don't say it. Instead of invalidating them, you can say something like, "*I am sorry about your loss. I'll always be here to listen when you are ready to talk.*"

"**Don't worry. You'll get pregnant again soon.**"

You are not acknowledging the pain they are feeling right now. It's okay that you want them to feel hopeful, but this phrase could be misinterpreted as dismissive. You may be completely wrong too. What if they have complications? What if the pregnancy loss led to more complicated issues or was caused by medical problems they are now aware of? What if the doctor gave them sad news after the pregnancy loss? You can instead say, "*this is hard. Would you like to talk about it?*"

"**Let me know if you need anything**."

This is a very kind, well-meaning statement. But when you are grieving, you barely have time to think about what you need or want. Offer to help them instead. You can say something like, "*oh, I'll drive by this week and bring you dinner. Which night would be okay?*"

"**You now know you can get pregnant.**"

It's good that you are trying to give them hope for the future, but there is nothing positive about this kind of loss. Speaking to someone who's experienced a loss is hard and can make anyone uncomfortable. You may be tempted to divert into something more positive and future-oriented. You may think this gives a sense of control in an otherwise hopeless situation. However, acting like they'd want to have another kid because they now know they can get pregnant is assumptive. You are assuming she would be interested in having other children in the future.

"*I understand how you feel*."

No, you don't. As I have said throughout this book, every pregnancy loss is different. Even if you've lost a child, your experience may differ. Everyone deals with grief uniquely. All they need is support and a listening ear. It's okay to admit that you are in no place to help them as much as you would like.

"*They are an angel now, looking down on you from heaven*" or **"*heaven needed another angel*."**

Ask anyone who's lost someone if they'd rather have an angel looking down on them or the person they've just lost. Many will choose the latter. They'd rather have their child here than an angel looking down on them. Maybe the person isn't religious or spiritual, so they don't believe there is an afterlife. Regardless of beliefs, most still prefer to have the baby with them.

Saying nothing

With such a long list of things you shouldn't say, you are probably wondering if you should just keep quiet. No, you shouldn't. Keeping quiet is worse and will only be awkward. Silence is one of the most dismissive and painful methods of communication. Even worse, it could be misinterpreted as ignoring them, you don't care, you are unavailable, or you don't notice them.

How do you handle some of these hurtful comments and cliches?

It's not always that people are trying to be hurtful or insensitive. It's just that some people don't know what to say to someone who's grieving and may even be uncomfortable around grief. Their intentions may be to comfort you, but they end up hurting you. With this in mind, you can handle the hurtful comments with grace. Decide that you'll forgive them in advance, even when they are insensitive or ignorant. Look beyond their words and examine their intent. Consider your relationship with them to understand their motive.

Many people will not know what to say, especially those who've never experienced pregnancy loss. It's not in your place to educate them about what they should and shouldn't say, but you can be prepared and respond with facts when someone says something insensitive, ignorant, or hurtful. I must tell you, though, it's easier to let it go and move on instead of getting into a confrontation with them. It's enough that you are dealing with something they don't understand.

If you must, respond with facts. Keep a cool head, but tell them when they are wrong. Here are some things you can say:

- Studies show that 10-25% of pregnancies could be lost through miscarriage, not to mention stillbirths.

- No one is to blame for a miscarriage, not even me. There are many reasons why pregnancies are lost, many of which we'll never know. Even experts who've studied pregnancy loss don't have all the facts.

- Grief is grief. Pregnancy loss is a loss, just like any other, and it's okay to mourn the loss of someone no matter the length of time.

Be blunt where necessary and set the record straight, especially when someone comes across as accusatory or when they are blaming you for the loss.

Sometimes, you don't feel like they are worth the effort. You don't feel the need to correct, educate or prove yourself to some people. Also, some people must win an argument and don't like being corrected. It's important to talk about what you feel, but it's better to talk to people who understand and listen. Change the conversation if you find that you need to prove yourself again and again.

Say something like:

- Maybe we can talk about something else?

- Right now, I'm not prepared to discuss this loss.

- Sorry, but I don't feel the need to discuss this.

Alternatively, you can change the subject altogether. You don't need to relive your experience to accommodate the other person.

You can also avoid people who don't understand. I know this may not always be practical or even possible, but choose your company wisely where you can. For example, if you know your mother-in-law is rude and insensitive and will probably offer insensitive, unsolicited advice, you can find excuses to avoid her. If possible, ask someone to intervene. It could be your partner. Your partner can warn them against making inappropriate, intrusive, or obnoxious comments. Forewarning the insensitive person to avoid the topic can save everyone a lot of heartache.

Three

Make Space for Grief

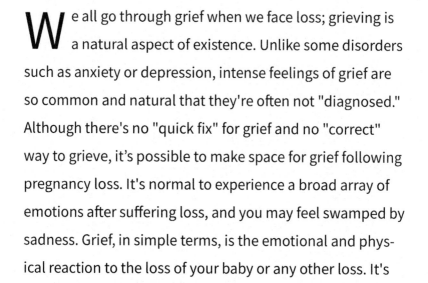

We all go through grief when we face loss; grieving is a natural aspect of existence. Unlike some disorders such as anxiety or depression, intense feelings of grief are so common and natural that they're often not "diagnosed." Although there's no "quick fix" for grief and no "correct" way to grieve, it's possible to make space for grief following pregnancy loss. It's normal to experience a broad array of emotions after suffering loss, and you may feel swamped by sadness. Grief, in simple terms, is the emotional and physical reaction to the loss of your baby or any other loss. It's accompanied by intense sadness and sorrow and frequently by a strong desire to see or be with your child.

Physical symptoms of grief include difficulties sleeping or eating and nausea. You might experience these emotions in waves, being tossed from one to the next. All these emotions are normal during the grieving process. Despite the discomfort, the grief process is crucial and necessary for healing.

Experiencing the pain of the loss

Every family member feels the impact of pregnancy loss because it is a traumatic and terrible occurrence that alters their lives and frequently leaves them with an overwhelming sense of emptiness. For the mother, the emotions are over the top. However, various stages of child loss, grief, and coping mechanisms might assist you and your family. There isn't a right or incorrect way to deal with the loss of a child, and giving yourself and other members of the family time to grieve is essential.

Further, it's important to remember that grieving varies from person to person; everybody has a unique way of grieving. Some people experience an array of emotions that overwhelm them, including astonishment, despair, denial, guilt, and fury. Others may feel sick, with symptoms including headaches, nausea, loss of appetite, insomnia, exhaustion, and difficulty concentrating. Again, some people cannot cry even though they feel they should. Some may even take months before they begin to feel "normal" and can resume their typical activities. The baby's due date and the anniversaries of the miscarriage may trigger severe grief.

Many parents worry that their physical and emotional responses to their partner's grieving aren't the same. This may be very challenging if you believe your partner doesn't care or understand what has happened. When experiencing intense grief and loss, it may not be easy to maintain a healthy relationship. However, it's crucial to have deep conversations, talking honestly and openly about your feelings and what you both need now. Listening is also vital; while this may be challenging, it will gradually get easier. Speaking with other friends, family, or professional support may be helpful when you and your spouse cannot meet each other's support needs (see chapter 4).

Because children's reactions to death differ significantly from those of adults, it's often difficult to predict how they will be affected. A toddler may be sad one moment and then appear okay and ready to play the next. Children use play to comprehend and make sense of the world around them. Children's grief may manifest in their behavior; some may become more demanding or uneasy, while others may become hostile or disruptive.

Your family and friends may show different reactions to your loss. They can be upset and unsure of how to support you. Sometimes they are speechless or will say things that you find cruel and accusatory. Other friends and relatives can be incredibly supportive in the first few weeks but expect you to quickly return to your typical routine. This can be unpleasant, and you may find that you need to tell them that life is very challenging for you at this point. Professional support groups can assist and offer information you can share with your family and friends.

Be gentle with yourself because losing a child can make you feel like your entire world is imploding. Furthermore, there may be feelings of disorientation, despair, and unfathomable sadness. No parent can be ready for the loss of their child. You must, therefore, give yourself space and practice self-compassion. Be kind to yourself as you would another person going through this. Be fair to yourself while you go through all the emotions associated with loss. It's quite acceptable to experience or go through the stages of mourning with difficulty. You may grieve in different ways; for example, talking about the lost child frequently may help you process the pregnancy loss and make sense of what you are going through.

Practice self-love and self-care. You'll be emotionally, intellectually, and physically worn out from grieving the death of a child, which is why self-care is important. When grieving feels all-consuming, it's easy to disregard your medical needs.

Your health is still crucial at this time. Among grief's typical health adverse effects are:

- Low immune system.

- Increased blood pressure.

- High blood sugar levels (diabetes).

- Lack of sleep.

- Loss of appetite.

- Heartburn.

As mentioned, grief can be physically taxing. Physical exercise can help. It is a common component of Cognitive-Behavioral Therapy (CBT) programs. This form of therapy has a positive effect on your body and mind. Exercise generates endorphins in the body, which will help break the loop of grieving-related thoughts, bodily sensations, hormones, and behaviors. Indeed, intense grief can be so overwhelming that you even struggle to get out of bed. It's okay if you feel like you can't do it. But getting out and walking in nature can help you think, clear your head, and put everything into perspective. You don't have to run miles or visit the gym if you don't want to. But I would encourage you to start small. Aim for short, basic bursts of movement throughout the day, and don't criticize your abilities or body.

Find what makes you feel happy. You can boost your physical activity by:

- Taking a walk.

- Stretching.

- Doing simple yoga.

The bottom line:

1. Don't just isolate yourself with your emotions.

2. Spend time with people who have experienced child loss because they can relate to your situation.

3. Allow other family members to cope with emotions in their ways.

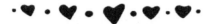

The lost dreams and grieving for what could have been; the ways men/women and children grieve.

Losing a child affects everyone differently. Even if feelings like grief, helplessness, and anger may be identical, how each individual interprets and expresses them varies considerably. Numerous elements influence how a person feels and communicates their sadness. Individual responses can vary depending on coping mechanisms, experiences in life, communication preferences, personality traits, and social support networks. Factors like gender and culture can also influence the way that people grieve. These elements affect how people process and communicate their emotions.

Although stereotypes don't apply to everyone, men and women frequently react to loss differently. However, acknowledging and promoting individual differences is more crucial than considering whether an emotion is more typical for a male or female. As they grow up, most men are taught to suppress their feelings. For them, crying is thought of and seen as a sign of weakness. People who'd like to be seen as tough and self-sufficient may restrain their emotions or refrain from discussing their pain.

During grief, men are likely to do the following:

- Not bringing up their loved one's death in a conversation. Many guys avoid painful conversations, which is how they cope with losing a loved one.

- Feel guilty for being unable to save their child from dying.

- Desire to overcome the loss rather than display sorrow. Some guys may have a desire to continue living their lives.

- Instead of seeking help, they try to handle grief by themselves.

- Unlikely to cry.

Men may try to cope by:

- **Engaging in strenuous or repetitive activities -** Some men may engage in physical activity, manual labor, yard work, or other pursuits as a diversion or release.

- **Additional work** - Though the desire to boost the family's financial security may be a factor, working more might also be a necessary diversion from negative emotions like loss and suffering.

- **Taking charge of family requirements** - Many fathers feel obligated to look after family members after a kid dies. They may accomplish this by taking responsibility for the finances, preparing arrangements for the burial, or taking over home tasks.

- **Sharing experiences and activities with family members** - Men may find it difficult to express grief. Many will try to bond with loved ones by engaging in activities together.

- **Becoming antisocial -** Some men isolate themselves and seek privacy as they go through the grieving process. They could become irate if they're not left alone.

Women, unlike men, are likely to share their pain with others. They are more open to making connections and accepting assistance from others.

During grief, women are likely to:

- **Make an effort to socialize** – Most women believe

that talking about their child loss experience helps in the healing process.

- Become irritated at other people's unwillingness to share their sadness.

- Break down in tears.

- Become restless.

- Experience loss of appetite and lack of sleep.

Women may attempt to cope by:

- **Frequently talking** about their losses with friends and family to handle their emotions.

- **Seeking assistance** - When grieving, women are more likely to seek support inside and outside the family than males.

- **Building brand-new** social networks. Grieving women may connect with people in their social circles or forge new ones, especially those who can relate to their sense of loss.

- **Interrogating or accusing others** - If a couple cannot discuss their loss and find solace in each other, some women may start to doubt their spouse or partner.

- **Writing about one's sorrow** - reading and writing novels, stories, or journals may encourage some women to interact with their inner selves and lessen their feelings of loneliness.

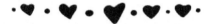

The 5 Stages of Grief

You'll probably go through all five grieving phases after pregnancy loss. The typical spectrum of feelings includes astonishment, rage, despair, and numbness. Anything you're feeling is acceptable. Everyone responds to pregnancy loss uniquely, and most miscarriage grief expressions are natural. Some people experience each of these stages sequentially, while others only go through a few, and yet more people experience the phases in a different order. It will be easier to comprehend what you're going through if you know what to anticipate.

Of the five stages of grief, we'll focus on depression and anxiety:

Depression after miscarriage or stillbirth

It's common to experience intense sadness and loss following pregnancy loss. These intense feelings can lead to clinical depression, and in some cases major depressive disorder, MDD. It's a mental condition that results in prolonged, severe, and persistent feelings of melancholy and despair.

For an accurate diagnosis of depression, you must have at least five of the symptoms listed below daily for at least two weeks:

- Sadness, emptiness, or hopelessness.

- Being irritable.

- Losing fun or interest in the majority of your routine activities.

- Feeling particularly exhausted and lacking energy.

- Getting either too little or too much sleep.

- Eating in excess or too little.

- Having apprehension, agitation, or anxiety.

- Feeling guilty or unworthy.

- Having issues with concentration, memory, and decision-making.

- Suicidal thoughts.

- Frequent aches that don't go away with treatment.

Depression after a pregnancy loss affects more than just the woman who experienced it. Researchers have found that a sizable proportion of men become depressed following their partner's pregnancy loss. Nevertheless, males typically bounce back from despair following the loss faster than women do. Studies show that women can struggle with depression long after the loss. Symptoms of depression can last a few weeks, months, or years, but many will recover from it within a year. Symptoms are typically effectively reduced by treatment, and a solid support system can assist women in getting back on their feet. Many women who experience pregnancy loss will go on to have healthy pregnancies.

In addition, you can find resources to assist you in overcoming depression following the loss of a baby. If you require assistance, don't be reluctant to ask for it. In chapter 7, we'll go into greater detail regarding managing depression.

Anxiety

Women frequently experience despair or anxiety symptoms after having a stillbirth or miscarriage. While most of us clearly know what depression is, many individuals mistakenly believe that anxiety is the same as "being on edge." However, there is more to anxiety than that. Like depression, anxiety can significantly impair a person's capacity to function. To properly overcome the underlying trauma, treatment and counseling are frequently necessary. In fact, the majority of studies report that anxiety disorders are more prevalent than depression following pregnancy loss.

Anxiety disorders are severe mental illnesses that result in persistently high levels of concern or fear that may potentially get worse with time. There are various kinds of anxiety disorders, each with unique characteristics.

The types of anxiety disorders commonly seen after pregnancy loss are:

Generalized Anxiety Disorders (GAD) - By definition, GAD is characterized by intrusive, excessive, and persistent concern that lasts longer than six months. The normal feelings of sadness that a woman may experience simply serve to intensify those anxieties. GAD is challenging to manage and can present with various symptoms, such as fatigue, muscle aches, poor concentration, and irritability.

Acute Stress Disorder (ASD) - One in ten women who have lost a pregnancy are thought to suffer from acute stress disorder. A traumatic incident is directly linked to ASD, which can appear hours after the occurrence. Contrary to popular belief, the time of pregnancy loss has no bearing on the risk of ASD. Studies show that women who've lost a pregnancy in the second trimester are more likely to experience ASD than those who've experienced a stillbirth in the third trimester.

Post-Traumatic Stress Disorder (PTSD) – Previous research shows that after losing a pregnancy, about 1% of women with ASD will develop post-traumatic stress disorder. In general, PTSD symptoms are similar to those of ASD, but they continue for more than a month. However, recent studies present a much different picture and contend that the prevalence of PTSD may be much greater. Furthermore, there is no correlation between the degree or kind of pregnancy loss experienced and the intensity of the PTSD symptoms.

Obsessive-Compulsive Disorder (OCD) – You may be intrigued to learn that obsessive-compulsive disorder, a con-

dition that experts think is influenced by hormones, is frequently encountered during pregnancy. On the other hand,
women who have lost a pregnancy have an eight-fold increased risk of being diagnosed with OCD. Obsessions with
excessive thoughts or ruminations, together with or without
compensating compulsive behaviors, are the hallmarks of
OCD. The unsettling thoughts could be aggressive and may
exacerbate the underlying anxiousness. OCD is frequently assumed to involve repetitive behaviors, although many
women merely suffer intrusive compulsions without the be-
havioral aspect.

Self-blame

Self-blame is among women's most prevalent emotions after pregnancy loss, along with guilt for the baby's death.
Self-blame leads to lingering emotions of ineptitude and
hesitation to try again out of dread of another loss. Most
women believe their pregnancies ended due to unplanned
pregnancy or because they had anxieties or uncertainties
about becoming mothers. Similar self-blame tendencies
also exist in men, although they manifest more strongly in
women.

Women are constantly subjected to societal messages about
how they should behave, look, and be treated. Both overtly

and covertly, they receive instructions on what to eat, drink, move, pluck, tuck, boost, and pose. If women deviate from the increasingly strict "standard," they are judged harshly. Some expectations on how to "behave" and act during pregnancy are conflicting. Different people and sources give conflicting instructions on what to drink, eat, and engage in to safeguard their unborn child. This makes it harder to have a "correct pregnancy," and you may blame yourself when things go wrong.

One further psychological fact, however, is unavoidable: mothers naturally desire to shield their kids from harm and always feel guilty if they cannot do so. A woman experiencing post-pregnancy loss grief also experiences the loss of potential, albeit strongly present, kid in her mind. Many people are unaware of the mother's true bond with the child because they don't see it physically.

Men and miscarriage

Uncertainty regarding a man's paternity may result after miscarriage. Before their children are even born, men can recognize that they are fathers and that their babies are real, thanks to ultrasounds. Men picture themselves as fathers when they see baby movements during pregnancy. This intense knowledge that the child is alive helps cement feelings of parenthood.

Unlike women, most men struggle with the idea of seeing themselves as fathers after a miscarriage. It may be challenging for them to mourn their paternity. Whether it was a miscarriage in the first trimester or because of the wrong idea that a fetus is not a human being, society frequently fails to acknowledge a miscarriage as a legitimate death. The repression of emotions can have a detrimental effect on a man's mental health and may lead to feelings of hopelessness and trouble coping. Men are more likely to experience delayed repercussions, according to studies.

Men are always torn between supporting their partners and expressing their grief. Many believe their emotions are valid given the situation even if they didn't experience the physical impact of pregnancy loss like the woman did. Still, most men choose the former - to support their partner and ignore their emotions. Societal expectations and their sense of obligation may be the primary causes of this behavior.

Following a miscarriage, women are allowed extra time and space to grieve, and their male partners offer support. Men can finally express their sorrow after women feel better and even then, they aren't offered as much help or support. Because males' contribution to pregnancy has historically been undervalued, their mourning is rarely accepted or seen as legitimate. Most men don't feel their loss is acknowledged. Furthermore, they feel the community doesn't provide the necessary space to grieve.

Additionally, due to the rarity of employers providing paid time off following a miscarriage, most men return to work once the pregnancy is lost. The disregard for giving dads time to digest their loss and the invalidity of fetal loss in social situations further create disenfranchised anguish.

Remembering the baby as a way to deal with grief

You'll probably be grieving the loss of your child, their lost future, and how your future will be. Finding a means to honor the loss may be helpful as the grieving process can be quite painful. You have the freedom to celebrate your child however you choose. Memorials are a great way to honor your lost child and express your love and grief. The term "memorial" originates from The Latin word "memos," meaning "mindful." As a result, memorials allow you to keep the child's memory with you in various ways.

Even if you never got to see, touch, or hug your baby, you can still make cherished memories of them. Use creative methods to honor your infant in your memory.

You can:

- Gather anything that will help you remember your child, such as clothes, toys, and ultrasound images, and put them in a scrapbook or a special container. These kinds of mementos may help you grieve your child.

- Give to a charity in your baby's honor, volunteer there, or provide a gift to a less fortunate youngster or pregnant woman. Create a project to honor your child, such as soliciting funds to erect a swing set in a public space.

- Have a funeral or a memorial service in honor of your infant. A memorial ceremony might provide you the opportunity to express sorrow and say goodbye to the child.

- Plant a tree to honor your child.

- Write feelings and thoughts down in a journal, or express them to your child in letters or poems. Let your infant know how you're feeling and how much they mean to you.

- Light candles or say prayers in memory of your infant on noteworthy occasions, such as the day the child passed on.

Dealing with anger

After losing a child, many women experience anger. Feelings of abandonment, guilt, the severity of the sorrow, the fact that their life has changed, the difficulty in grieving, and the abrupt sense of the world feeling empty, dangerous, or lonely all contribute to anger. There may be instances when you have sudden eruptions of fury while going through the grieving process. It frequently comes as an unannounced and unwanted reaction that just happens. Maybe there's someone, in particular, you're mad at. You could be angry with your lost child or the person you think caused the loss, such as the doctor, your partner, or even yourself. Even close relatives and friends have the potential to offend you by acting or saying things that you may find annoying.

Sometimes you may not even have a specific reason or target on your mind; you may just feel angry with everyone. You may be in pain and frustrated because you don't know why you lost your baby, and the unfairness makes you want to shout. You may have directed your anger more broadly at "fate," life, or even God for permitting the loss. You may occasionally feel purely enraged!

Anger is a common response to grief and sadness; having periodic fits of rage is acceptable. However, if you allow anger to fester for too long, it will become a more powerful emotion of wrath, which can spiral out of control. Unresolved anger can lead to bitterness. Anger can also develop into fury and vengeance if it's allowed to simmer for too long. These are unwelcome by-products of a typical feeling that are harmful and damaging. Your current anger will eventually disappear, but only through patience and forgiveness. Although the energy is still present, you can allow your anger to transform from destructive to positive.

Before it's fully resolved, anger frequently ebbs and flows. Yes, rage can be dealt with, and it ought to be. You have the option to let go of the potent and destructive emotion of anger rather than keep it inside of you for an extended period. If you hold onto it for too long, your healing process will be much longer. Even though having these feelings is common, it's crucial to express them. As angry as you may be, never vent, project, or make someone feel like it's their fault.

You can do some things to manage your anger and let these feelings out productively. When you're angry:

- Slowly count to ten or take a few long, deep breaths.

- Use art forms such as drawing and painting to express your rage.

- Speak with a member of your support network or express all of your feelings in a notebook. Don't worry about sounding "correct," just be honest and transparent when you describe what makes you furious.

- You can release the negative energy through movement and exercise.

- You could feel like physically expressing your feelings; sometimes, fury cannot be expressed in words. Find a private space or area to express yourself during those times by yelling, stomping your feet, kicking, moving around violently, shaking your body, banging your fists against a pillow, or running. However, if you decide to do so, tell someone you trust what you're doing. Always take safety precautions too. Never let your wrath get the better of you or cause harm to others.

- You could decide to channel the negative energy into something positive by taking up activism for a particular cause or supporting change where it's necessary.

- Scribble furiously or tear off strips of scrap paper, wad them all up, and toss them in the garbage, then imagine your rage being dumped with the paper.

You may discover that talking about your emotions and lending a hand to others brings happiness. Decide to let all anger out and substitute it with love.

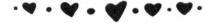

Four

Find Support

♥

We typically anticipate help from close relatives after a family member passes away. However, miscarriage is peculiar in that you may choose to grieve alone or seek support from people who understand pregnancy loss, but who are not part of the family. If a person had a miscarriage or stillbirth and handled the situation well, their comfort and reassurance can be invaluable. One of the underlying and universal themes among women who suffer pregnancy loss is the feeling that they are so alone in the pain. Support is essential to navigate the trauma of the loss. But before we take a deep dive deeper into the benefits of support, let's break down the numbers to illustrate just how frequently pregnancy loss happens. The fact that it is so common does not diminish your pain. These facts are only shared to let you know you absolutely are not alone. Miscarriage happens in all countries, in all ethnic groups, all ages, all socioeconomic situations.

The statistics

Estimates vary, but March of Dimes, a group that promotes mother and child health, reports between 10 and 15 percent of miscarriages among women with confirmed pregnancy. Around the world, pregnancy loss is characterized in different ways. But in general, a baby who passes away before the beginning of the third trimester is called a miscarriage, and babies who pass away at or beyond 28 weeks are stillbirths. Many of the almost 2 million stillbirths that occur each year are avoidable. Substantially in affluent nations, stillbirths and miscarriages are rarely routinely reported, indicating that the actual incidences may be even higher.

The number of miscarriages and stillbirths can be decreased in several ways. This includes expanding access to prenatal care (in some parts of the world, women don't see a health care provider until they are several months pregnant), establishing a continuum of care via midwife-led care, and, where practical, implementing community care. Moreover, most women who experience first-time miscarriages are unlikely to experience it again. The likelihood of miscarrying in your subsequent pregnancy is roughly 20%. The likelihood of another miscarriage is 28% if you've experienced two prior miscarriages. Also, if you've had a miscarriage three times, the likelihood of experiencing another miscarriage is 43%. If you've experienced two or more miscarriages, testing for the causes of the miscarriages may be helpful.

Most pregnancies end in miscarriage for reasons the woman can't change or control. Genetic problems are a significant contributor to miscarriages early in pregnancy. These genetic problems mean the child couldn't have lived outside the womb. Even with this kind of pregnancy loss, a woman can still become pregnant and give birth to a healthy baby in the future without any problems. Early in the development process, when fetuses are most sensitive, other factors, including obesity or malnutrition, can have the most detrimental impact. That's why most miscarriages happen in early pregnancy.

Here is a general breakdown of miscarriage risk by week:

3rd to 4th week

Implantation typically occurs a week after ovulation and three weeks after the last menstruation. A home pregnancy test might reveal a positive result by week 4. Sadly, up to 50 to 75% of pregnancies end before a pregnancy test shows a positive result. Though some women may have suspicions due to pregnancy loss symptoms, most won't know they were pregnant.

5th week

At this stage, the miscarriage rate varies considerably. Research shows a 21.3% probability of losing a pregnancy after the 5th week.

6th to 7th week

According to the same study, the loss percentage lowers to 5% after week 6. During this period, it's typically possible to see a heartbeat on an ultrasound.

8th to 13th week

The rate of miscarriage appears to be between two and four percent in the 2nd half of the first trimester.

14th to 18th week

The likelihood of miscarriage during this period is less than 1%. However, stillbirth is still a real risk. A stillbirth might induce labor in some people. Because of contemporary technology, very small newborns may be able to live outside the womb, making stillbirths relatively uncommon around the 14th to 18th week.

Risk of miscarriage by age

Age is a significant risk factor for pregnancy loss. The age factor can be attributed to the deteriorating egg quality over time. According to a woman's age, the typical likelihood of miscarriage is as follows:

- Below 35 years – 15% chance of miscarriage.

- 35-45 years – 20-35% likelihood of miscarriage.

- Above 45 years – 50% chance of miscarriage.

It's crucial to remember that these statistics are averages and don't account for any other factors. Age can also be compounded by the negative impacts of lifestyle choices, like smoking or living a sedentary lifestyle. This could exacerbate existing medical conditions and raise the possibility of miscarriage. Despite this, some women experience a safe pregnancy in their 40s, and a small number do so in their 50s.

Does cigarette smoking (active or passive) increase the risk of miscarriage?

Well, yes. The risk of miscarriage is increased by tobacco usage and cigarette smoking. The likelihood of miscarriage increases as a woman smokes more. According to studies, each daily cigarette smoked by a woman increases her rela-

tive risk of miscarriage by 1%. Quitting smoking can significantly increase the likelihood of having a healthy pregnancy.
Women who've quit smoking can carry a pregnancy to term
just as well as those who have never smoked. Also, the risk
of miscarriage is increased by secondhand smoking —up to
11%.

How about taking alcohol?

Regular alcohol consumption during the first trimester of
pregnancy raises the risk of miscarriage. A 2014 San Francis-
co research of 1,061 women found that women who drank
spirits (as opposed to wine or beer) and those who consumed four or more alcoholic beverages per week had a
higher chance of miscarriage. The risk of child loss also increases with the consumption of illegal substances such as
heroin, opioids, cocaine, and methamphetamine.

As we've seen above, miscarriage is common. So, you're not
alone. Thus, don't be too hard on yourself. Beating yourself
up by saying that you're cursed or have bad luck will only
worsen things. Having these statistics in mind will help you
combat misconceptions. Understanding that drugs increase
the risk of a miscarriage is an excellent start. If you take
alcohol or smoke, you may want to consider quitting for a
while until after your baby is here.

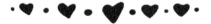

Reaching out for support

Since the grief caused by loss can lead to detachment and isolation, it's necessary to stress the importance of getting assistance from others to heal. Even though support is essential for healing, many people struggle with and find it uncomfortable to express their emotions. Sharing your feelings over losing someone can be comforting, but this doesn't mean that every conversation you have with family or friends has to center on that particular loss.

Being surrounded by your loved ones might provide you comfort. Besides friends and family, you can express your sorrow in a support group where people who have experienced a similar situation gather. Alternatively, you can get therapy from a doctor or therapist qualified to assist their patients in resolving their complex emotions and getting back on their feet after a loss.

Given your body's increased hormone production, the agony of grieving, and the sense that your entire world has suddenly been utterly destroyed, you might not think as clearly as you usually would. Please keep the following in mind while reaching out to family, friends, and coworkers for support:

- **Decide on the timing**. The other person's mental health is equally important. They may be too busy, struggling themselves, or the timing might not be right. It's preferable to do it in person whenever you can. Don't use anyone to reach out on your behalf because you're unlikely to receive the comfort and support you desire. Also, break the news about your miscarriage in a serene environment such as your home. Keep in mind that they, too, will be shocked.

- **Pick your support circle wisely**. Your friends may be unfamiliar with pregnancy loss and what you feel, so they don't realize that it's the most significant event in your life. Unfortunately, despite their best intentions, they'll probably feel the need to comment, even though they're aware that nothing they can say will help you feel better. Because silence is worse, they may try making up for it by saying things you find hurtful or dismissive.

I would recommend support groups and close, supportive family members and loved ones. They can help you in various ways, but they may focus their efforts on three fundamental goals. The three objectives of these support groups will help you:

- **Embrace hope**. The people around you give you hope even when you feel cut off from the things that make life worthwhile. They can help you through this trying period and give you hope that you will recover.

- **Face the reality of your loss**. These folks know your desire to reflect on and express your sorrow. They give you a safe space to publicly grieve and assist you in "telling your tale." In essence, they extend an invitation for you to express the pain you are feeling outside of yourself.

- **Have "companions" along the journey**. These people act as companions who can validate your sorrow. They know genuine compassion stems from "walking with" someone rather than going before or after them. To "carry a heavy weight" is what the verb "grieve" means. Those that support you during your grief are aware that by doing so, they give you optimism that something positive will come from your sadness.

The people closest to you are there to offer support and companionship. They are aware of your feelings and what you're going through. So, ensure you take advantage of this opportunity or actively seek them out.

Coping with hurtful words

Everyone likes to keep the conversation going, but knowing the right things to say or do while someone is mourning can be challenging. As a result, the majority turn to typical cliches in the hope that they will provide some solace and relief.

Although most people have good intentions, they sometimes use clichés out of concern that they would say something inappropriate. Besides, nobody is naturally gifted with the ability to understand what to tell a person grieving the loss of a loved one. In general, people avoid having dialogues about death and sorrow.

You may typically be adept at disregarding critical remarks. Laughing it off can help you handle people and distressing remarks. However, the depth of the loss can make even well-intended comments feel cruel, and, regrettably, there are situations when people may not even be aware they have wounded you. Others may have negative opinions regarding the circumstances of your child's death. Others may say that the child's death is good because that's "nature's way."

In other instances, grief leads you to mistakenly believe that a friend or relative is criticizing or disparaging you when they are not. When you are grieving, your emotions are so strong that even the tiniest comments you may have ignored in another situation can devastate you.

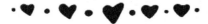

How to cope

There are several methods to handle situations where someone has said something unpleasant to you or is acting in a disrespectful way. Consider the best course of action for you, and never forget that this sadness is yours and that you should be permitted to experience it in its whole.

- **Practice letting it go. Forgive.**

Is the argument worth the time and effort? Maybe a loved one who said something upsetting in passing didn't intend it.

You already feel a myriad of emotions in your grief. Is it really worth your time and energy directly confronting someone about a trivial remark? So, sometimes it's best to let it go. Even if you think they're wrong, it might be wiser to put your mental health and your energy first and forgive their wrong-doing. Forgiveness does not mean you excuse the remark and say "it's okay" they hurt you. Forgiveness comes from compassion and frees you up to let go of the comment and the hurt attached to it so that you don't keep looping around it and replaying the story and reliving the pain.

- **Inform them strongly and plainly that their actions are not helpful**

Tell someone boldly and without fear that their remarks are adding to the pain of grieving if they repeatedly say unpleasant things and won't be convinced to stop. Despite what they think, you are allowed to express your pain because it's real.

- **Spend time with people who are grieving**

Spend quality time with other understanding family members and friends. Although it's not necessary, it might be comforting to know that your loved ones at least somewhat get what you're going through.

- **If anything upsets you, open up**

If a close friend or family member continually uses a term that distresses you, open up and tell them how offending it is. For instance, if they say, "everything happens for a reason," you may respond by saying, "I know you don't intend to upset me, but I find such comments unhelpful." They may be unaware of how their comments are affecting you. If you are honest with them, they'll know what to say and what not to say.

- **Stay away from negative people**.

It's okay to stay away from someone if their actions bring you great distress regularly. Perhaps you might rekindle your friendship in the future when your sadness is less acute. However, right now, you only need as many encouraging and understanding voices as you can find, not critical ones.

- **Join a support group**

There are lots of support groups, especially online, that focus on child loss. This implies that the group members will be aware of the societal prejudices you are fighting against, at least to some extent. Sharing your pregnancy loss experience with others in similar situations might be a significant step toward healing.

You may wish to seek more assurance and direction if you feel that particular comments or attitudes are seriously upsetting you or if you're unable to stop thinking about something that was said.

For professional guidance on navigating grief and the reactions of others around you, consider getting in touch with a specialized bereavement support organization.

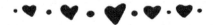

Finding medical support

You may wonder, "*When does 'natural' grief become an issue requiring expert assistance?*" Most of the time, a loss can be harrowing and disorienting, making it challenging to imagine how to continue living. Other times, you may feel like you're not reacting particularly strongly and wonder if you should. Following a loss, it's common for women to believe they're "going insane." Given enough time and compassionate support, grief can eventually result in profound contemplation and growth, no matter how difficult it may seem.

If you experience persistent functioning deficits (interpersonal issues, workplace issues, or trouble performing crucial duties), then it's time to seek counseling or therapy. You may benefit from counseling if you're going through any of the following:

- **Insufficient social support**. While friends and family can be a terrific support system through trying times, there comes a time in your life when you have no one or are left with few people to turn to. A counselor can offer additional assistance, delivering sincere compassion and company through the trying moments. By recommending bereavement groups, they can keep you in touch with other grieving people.

- **Sleep disruptions**. Consistent sleep problems, such as difficulty falling asleep, waking up throughout the night, or oversleeping, can interfere with your energy, mood, and focus, making it challenging to take care of the obligations and relationships important to you. You can create routines that will encourage a long and peaceful night's sleep with the assistance of a counselor.

- **Role changes or stress**. Your life may change due to the loss, forcing you to adapt or take on new responsibilities. For instance, you might discover that you need to shoulder more responsibilities for household management, child-rearing, or bill payment. After losing your baby, it can be challenging to maintain existing relationships or establish new ones. Counseling can help you manage stress, find workable solutions to the issues brought on by role shifts, and determine areas of your life where you can make a significant contribution.

Some other reasons may also make grieving more complicated, and it may seem appropriate to seek the assistance of a mental health expert. Find a qualified practitioner who practices evidence-based psychotherapy if you are experiencing any of the following:

- **Worry and grief**

Losing your child can cause a lot of anxiety. Without the child, life might seem strange and unsettling. You may lose the sense of security you had before, making you more conscious of your vulnerability and mortality. Despite this being a logical and normal response to loss, many people battle with worry. Working with a therapist might be beneficial for learning new coping mechanisms and expanding your viewpoint.

- **Complex or protracted grief**

It is typically true that bereaved individuals' functioning returns, even without counseling, given enough time and care. But according to research, 10% of bereaved women experience significant and long-lasting deficits in their functioning (some go longer than a year), in which case counseling may be helpful.

- **History of addiction**

Strong emotions may push someone to substance abuse, particularly those with a history of addiction. With the help of a therapist, develop effective emotional coping skills to help you make a decision that is more in line with your beliefs. Please feel free to contact qualified mental health specialists who can assist you in finding the support you require to cope with sorrow, loss, and any potential effects.

Expressing grief

There is no deeper human bond than that between mothers and their child(ren). Sadly, all parents must consider the prospect of losing this bond should their child pass away. Expressing your sorrow in public or private is a healthy component of mourning that can help you achieve closure after a loss. Grief rituals and cultural customs are frequently associated with how people express their grief publicly. Public funerals, memorial services, and burials are commonplace when a community stands with families who have lost a family member. Some people feel more at ease expressing their suffering in solitude, while others prefer getting support from their society.

These outward displays of grief are intended to have an impact, assist grieving individuals in their process, and relieve the emotional burden of grieving privately. The following advice may be helpful as you learn to deal with your loss and wish to express your sadness and pain openly:

- **Express your emotions**

A variety of emotional and physical experiences are typical of responses to mourning. It's important to express your sadness and loss in a way that seems genuine to you because everyone grieves in their unique way. Intense pain and suffering, irritation, rage, disorientation, and a host of other mourning reactions that may have been unfamiliar to you may come up during the grieving process. Letting out all your emotions will help you process your grief.

- **Speak to your loved ones**

Speaking with your family and support network is essential for the healing process. Being open with your support group members lets them know you appreciate their encouragement and care, especially when needed. Many people may avoid you until you have recovered from your loss because they are unsure of how to approach you during this time.

Some may feel uncomfortable discussing death, while others may be unsure of what to say. You can start the conversation by sharing stories with them about your child, how their passing has affected your life, and how you're coping with it.

- **Post on social media**

Posting on social media will let others know what you're experiencing. It is a thoughtful method to express your grief honestly and publicly. Most people will be eager to help you out, and knowing that there are people who care about you may be comforting during this time. Remember that you just need to provide the information that makes you feel comfortable; you're not required to share your loss's specifics. Think about limiting the audience for your content.

Support systems

Support groups are typically regarded as credible and reputable recommendations, and many say these groups have helped them cope with their sorrow. Besides the fact that they are widely accessible, typically cost nothing, and call for a little commitment from participants, grief support groups provide several potential advantages.

Here are examples of how support groups differ from one another:

- Culture and attitude.

- Structure.

- Peer-led rather than a mental health professional-led.

- It may be centered on specific loss as opposed to general.

- It is centered on advocacy and action as opposed to grieving.

Advantages of support groups

As we've already mentioned, support groups and those participating have distinct personalities. Here are some benefits.

Give hope

In a support group, those experiencing acute grief can interact with people far more advanced in their healing. Group leaders frequently have personal experience with loss. Those doing well in the group and discovering new forms of healing can give hope to those experiencing sadness for the first time and demonstrate that joy can be felt again.

Sharing knowledge

People who have gone through similar events may offer valuable insights, pieces of advice, beneficial suggestions, and understanding. While it's not mandatory to adopt all the advice given, it will enable you to fine-tune and understand your viewpoint and approach better because everyone copes with grief differently.

Universality

Being reminded that you're not alone is one of the best things about joining a grief support group. Grief can make you feel incredibly lonely and isolated, especially if no one nearby seems to be experiencing or understanding it. Attending a support group may help you discover that other people share your experiences, sentiments, and challenges. The support group network can be a shelter of understanding for you when you feel wholly alone and misunderstood by others.

Kindness

Offering assistance and gifts can be therapeutic. Members of support groups have the chance to provide and receive support and advice from one another. In your grief, you will discover a lot about who you are, your life, and other people; support groups give you the chance to share your knowledge with others. Until they find themselves assisting and supporting someone else through their grieving challenges, people frequently are unaware of how much they have to offer.

Cohesiveness

Everyone has a natural urge to fit in. Being a part of a community and experiencing acceptance and validation is satisfying. You realize just how important group membership can be when you contemplate how belonging may affect your happiness and how your child's death made you feel odd, lonely, and isolated. Nobody wants to be a member of the grief club, but once you are, there are many advantages to being around other members.

Disadvantages of support groups

Support groups have numerous benefits. However, they also have drawbacks:

Discouraging

People frequently go to support groups for advice, hope, and comfort. Those who are grieving for the first time, in particular, might be hoping for signs that things get better. You may feel hopeless when you learn that people in a group, especially those who are further along in their loss, are still expressing anguish, irritation, and negativity.

Therapeutic expectations

It's crucial to remember that support groups and therapy are two entirely different things. Some group leaders work in the mental health field; however, most do not. If you seek a more formal therapy approach, you might want to speak with a psychotherapist.

Misinformation

If it occurs at the grocery shop, why wouldn't it happen in a gathering of people who are all experiencing grief? You'll find that there are advantages to learning from others' experiences, but there can also be misinformation about what is typical, what to anticipate, and how to adapt.

Don't take suggestions too seriously, but if it works for you, terrific! If not, try to concentrate on taking something positive away from other people's experiences and finding strength in their encouragement.

Five

Loving Relationships

Grief is normal, a natural part of being human. Grief is complex; it takes time and may involve distinct emotions and behaviors. These emotions and behaviors are known as grief reactions. Grief reactions vary from one individual to the next and even within the same person during different times. These reactions commonly include burdensome emotions, thoughts, and behaviors. Everyone experiences and deals with grief emotions differently. Most of us will feel these emotions come in cycles of waves. This is to say that you may, at one moment, feel calm only to experience overwhelming, heartbreaking emotions a few minutes or hours later.

When you are calm, you may think you have your emotions in control and are making progress, when in reality, you may be in the "small wave" or "calm water" period. Soon after, the grief may overwhelm you again, making you feel like you are back where you started. This is completely normal. Most people admit that significant dates or events such as holidays and birthdays are powerful triggers for overwhelming grief emotions. Over time, some of these emotions may subside, and you may experience the grief emotions less frequently as you slowly adjust to the loss. With that said, it's important to understand that loss and grief are experienced differently by everyone. This understanding can help bring compassion and understanding to relationships that the trauma of loss can strain.

Pregnancy loss causes marital and relationship strain.

Pregnancy loss impacts many relationships around the grieving couple. Many couples also learn that their relationship also suffered and may have changed following the traumatic event. Results of a University of Michigan study showed that even though most couples become closer during and after pregnancy loss, many others grow apart, and their relationships take a huge blow. This negative impact of pregnancy loss on relationships was even more pronounced in couples already struggling before the miscarriage or stillbirth and in younger or cohabitating individuals.

Moreover, the researchers also observed that the support network around the grieving couple had a massive impact on those specific relationships following pregnancy loss. As I've said before, society doesn't acknowledge pregnancy loss like other losses. Even people close to the couple may not acknowledge it, and this can really put a strain on the relationship in question. Many people around the couple may be uncomfortable, while others may say rude, unhelpful, or ignorant things. By avoiding this issue, the grieving couple is left to cope with the loss themselves.

Even more complicated are the different ways the individuals in the relationship grieve following pregnancy loss and its impact on their relationship. The study showed that couples' relationships might suffer when they have different coping methods. Men and women grieve differently. For this reason, a couple may find themselves in conflict over the other person's coping mechanism. This is a volatile period in any couple's life, so the conflicts may only worsen the situation.

"Parents with significantly different grieving patterns may be at a particularly high risk for subsequent marital conflict or emotional withdrawal."

According to the study, couples dealing with the trauma of pregnancy loss, whether married or cohabiting, had a 22%

increased risk of breaking up than couples with live births. Sadly, the risk was established to be higher in couples who had a stillbirth. The study reports the risk of breaking up is 40% higher in couples that experienced a stillbirth. In comparison, a miscarriage impacted the first two or three years of a relationship, while the effect after stillbirths persisted for nearly ten years. With stillbirth, the couple may have bonded more with the child, chosen a name, probably knew the gender, and had already prepared for its arrival.

"Both mothers and fathers of stillborn children often have experienced the infant kicking and have heard fetal heart sounds. The anticipated birth is, therefore, more tangible to both parents."

Many couples experience relationship conflicts after a miscarriage or stillbirth, especially if they feel differently.

A study published by the journal *Psychosomatic Medicine* showed that for first-time fathers, the reality of fatherhood only starts to sink in when they first hold their babies in their arms. It's unsurprising then that a couple may deal with the loss differently. The woman may experience the loss more deeply because of the womb connection. The partner will grieve too, but they may desire normalcy sooner. The only reminder of the pregnancy to the partner is the sight of the mother who lost the pregnancy. On the contrary, the women felt the baby biologically daily. The baby was growing inside her.

Based on two open-ended questions, women who experienced pregnancy loss shared a lot about the impact of miscarriage and stillbirth on their relationships in a new study. The main focus of this study was:

- The effect of pregnancy loss on the relationship with the partner

- The impact of pregnancy loss on sexual relationships with their partner

28% of women who experienced pregnancy loss were pregnant again one year after the loss. Another 29% were trying again and hoping to get pregnant, while 34% were still grieving and were avoiding pregnancy altogether. While there wasn't much variation in the women's opinions about pregnancy, the same didn't apply to variations in relationships.

After pregnancy loss:

- 23% of women felt closer to their partners after pregnancy loss. On the contrary, only 6% thought they had a close sexual relationship with their partner.

- 44% of women felt that their relationship returned to the way it was before the pregnancy loss. 55% of the women thought that the sexual bond had returned to how it was before the pregnancy loss.

- 32% of women felt they didn't have the same relationship they had before the pregnancy. They felt distant from their partners. 39% of women also felt sexually distant from their partners.

Women who felt closer to their partners had more emotional strength and were more likely to be pregnant again. The same women felt their partners were supportive, actively sharing their loss and grief.

On the contrary, the women who'd grown distant from their partners reported more conflicts in their relationships. Many felt their partners weren't doing much to show if or when they cared. The women also agreed that they struggled with mental health issues, including tension, anger, confusion, anxiety, and depression. Many were angry at life, themselves, and their partners. Sadly, the women avoided sexual intimacy, had a lesser desire for it, and only had sex as a functional necessity. To them, sex was like a scary reminder of what they'd lost, a painful, heartbreaking memory. Some of the women also felt abandoned.

Most women felt understood and supported when their partners shared their feelings. It helped them deal with the difficulty of the situation and pull through the trauma. In short, the relationship is at great risk if the partner isn't responsive. The partner needs to be extra attentive to the woman. If the partner maintains open communication with the grieving mother, the relationship may thrive even after the pregnancy loss.

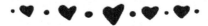

How men and women grieve differently and their roles for each other while grieving

Pregnancy loss causes trauma that some people never truly get over; they only learn to live with it. And as it is, everyone will grieve the loss differently, you, your partner, family, friends, and children, if you have any. Indeed, you and your partner may agree on a lot, but both of you may experience different emotions at different times and respond to them differently.

This may cause problems, as I have discussed above. You may feel angry thinking your partner isn't as upset about the pregnancy loss as they should be. You may feel abandoned or that they don't care that much. On the contrary, your partner may feel like you are too emotional and may not be supportive of how much you talk about the loss. Because you are the one who's showing emotions, he may be ignored. Loved ones may only be more concerned about you, asking how you are doing and ignoring him and his feelings.

Here's how you may express yourself after the loss:

- Talking about the pregnancy loss often and with everyone around you

- Crying a lot and frequently

- Feeling emotional often

- Asking people around for help

- Joining a support group

- Joining a church, mosque, or another place of worship.

Your partner may show his grief differently:

- Sitting and grieving alone

- Unlike you, he may not talk much about the miscarriage or stillbirth

- To keep his mind off the loss, he may resort to working extra hours or taking on additional hobbies, such as spending more time at the gym or hanging out with his friends

- He feels the loss but may not know how to express himself

- Some think that speaking up will make them look weak, or others may perceive them as weak when they do

- He may try to act strong and protective of the family as people expect him to

- Many won't ask for help. They'll find a way to work through the grief alone.

There is no rule or guidebook on how people should express or deal with grief. There is a good chance men and women will express grief in the different ways described above, but there isn't a one-size-fits-all way of expressing your sadness. It's okay to let people grieve the best way they know how. Be patient with each other and try talking about how you feel and how you'd like to remember your lost baby.

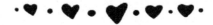

What about children?

Children feel sadness too. They also grieve and can sense when something is wrong. When your older children learn of the pregnancy loss, they may act out, act scared, or be in desperate need of attention and care. Many don't understand pregnancy loss, so some may think your life is in danger. Some children may be scared of losing you, while others may think they did something wrong and are to blame for losing their sibling. Even though they are young, children deal with grief better when they understand what's happening. Sit with them and explain everything as clearly as you can. Use simple anecdotes and honest words, so you don't scare them.

Here are a few illustrations of how you can help them understand the loss:

- For example, tell them, "The baby was too small. The baby was born tiny, and we couldn't bring him home." You'll only confuse them more if you say things like "I lost the baby" or "the baby is still sleeping."

- Read children's stories that explain death and loss in a way they can understand. You can find such books at your neighborhood library or funeral home. The stories will help you clarify what death is.

- Ask them how they feel about the loss if and when they understand it. Give them space to ask questions about how you are doing and what happened.

- If they can, ask them to give suggestions on how to remember the child. They may draw a picture, create a piece of art, or help them plant a tree in the child's memory.

- Explain that neither you nor them will die because of the loss. Let them know they aren't to blame for this; no one is.

Children hurt, just like the rest of us. They may feel angry, confused, and upset. You may notice that they are clingy or cranky if they are younger. They may also surprise you by acting in ways they haven't in so long. The older ones may appear worried. Some older children may appear unbothered and show no reaction to the loss. Others may ask questions that sound rude and ignorant. Be patient with them. Many only act out because they don't understand the gravity of the situation.

Alternatively, a grief counselor may help your older children process their grief and sadness. The grief counselor works directly with the children and can recommend valuable resources to help them overcome the loss.

It's not uncommon for male partners to experience feelings of grief of a similar intensity to women.

Research into pregnancy loss and the subsequent support services have always been focused on women. Indeed, multiple studies have shown that women struggle more with losing an anticipated future and their unborn children. Many women may struggle with their new identity after pregnancy loss, mainly if they are first-time mothers. In most cases, partners are the closest and primary support figures for grieving mothers. There is proof that a caring partner and a positive support system are crucial during this time. When a mother receives care and support from her partner, she is more likely to deal with the grief and distress of pregnancy loss better and may even recover faster.

Unfortunately, the same level of care, understanding, and support hasn't been extended to the male partner's experience following pregnancy loss. Very minimal research has been done in this area, and most people don't understand how men feel after this loss. Although men are likely to experience the same emotions, many admit that these feelings don't last as long as the women's and may not be as intense.

However, new research shows that following pregnancy loss, men may experience as much or even higher grief levels as the mother. Many men view themselves as protectors and supporters, affecting how they express their grief. Most deal with their grief privately and internally. Previous studies showed that men found distractions and used avoidance behavior to deal with grief. Societal expectations on how men should grieve, the lack of recognition of their suffering, and the assumption that all they should do is be supportive may be major contributing factors to this behavior.

Men also feel like their grief is devalued, not only by society, but also by support people, including healthcare professionals, hospital staff, therapists, and religious leaders. Many men feel left out, unsupported, and misunderstood. No one acknowledges their grief, and when they do, it's not in the same way as their female partners. Many men feel excluded and marginalized from support, information, and hospital care.

The limited research also indicates that men's emotional needs are more likely to be overlooked or completely ignored by their social networks. Moreover, men are reluctant to share their grief, so it's harder for friends and family to help, even when they are willing. Studies show that men also feel like they have few people to share their grief with and that society ignores them. Many men admit they are reluctant to share their problems with their social networks, arguing that the issue was too personal , out of respect for their partner's preferences, or that they may be judged or expected to have moved on. But society isn't to blame for everything.

Previous research has shown that generally, men seek medical help and other healthcare services less than women. These negative health-seeking behaviors have been linked to men's male identity and the outdated ideas of what mas-culinity should look like. These behaviors cut across cul-tures, countries, and age groups. Some of these traditional ideas associated with the men's identity include stoicism, which is the fear of appearing weak when they seek help. For this reason, many men would rather act independent and tough and endure pain even amid intense pain and great hardship. It's sad, but studies show that men who've adopt-ed these beliefs were more likely to smoke. They reportedly have a higher risk of physical injury caused by accidents and are more inclined to suffer from mental health prob-lems such as depression, anxiety, and dysfunctional coping mechanisms.

Even so, men still need emotional support following preg-nancy loss. They would appreciate formal support groups, counseling, and encouragement that sharing their grief with other men like brothers, fathers, and male friends is okay. This area of study needs more research if we are to under-stand how men experience pregnancy loss, how they ex-press their grief emotions after a miscarriage or stillbirth, the necessary emotional support, and how best to support them when it happens. Not only will this research help us understand men's experiences, but we'll also know how to be supportive and where to focus those efforts.

Men may feel helpless because men typically are fixers and problem solvers.

Many men feel helpless after a pregnancy loss. After all, they are programmed to protect, fix and solve problems. Understandably, your partner may feel obligated to try and fix the problem. Sadly, this isn't a problem they can fix; nobody can. Pregnancy loss isn't something we can control, no matter how powerful we are. They can't do much except support you and deal with their grief.

Other men may take on their role as protectors more seriously. They'll support their partner and fixate on daily tasks such as caring for older children, working, shopping, etc. This they do to try and make life easier for their grieving partners. This works when the man isn't overwhelmed by the loss, but they should also get the time, space, and necessary support to grieve.

Emotional isolation

A new study shows that pregnancy loss affects many relationships around a woman, not only with their partners but also with their extended families and friends. For example, some struggled in the company of other pregnant family members, colleagues, or others who'd recently given birth.

These feelings and emotions were sometimes misinterpreted by family members, which strained their relationships. Many women felt that their feelings of isolation, which were already present, had been exacerbated by this.

Friends and family who'd have been their source of support kept off because their presence reminded the women of their loss. Some women avoided certain functions – baby showers, pregnancy announcements, gender reveals, etc. Not only did this avoidance behavior increase family tension, but it also increased the women's sense of isolation. The isolation aggravated the grieving woman's loss and reduced the emotional support available for them during the grieving process.

Furthermore, there was a lack of understanding from loved ones about the extent and length of their grief. Some people were uncomfortable around them and cautious about everything they said. Others were at a loss of words; they didn't know what to say, so they avoided the topic altogether. Many women in the study described a level of grief that stretched beyond what their loved ones thought and felt appropriate. Not only were their social networks uncomfortable around this grief, but many couldn't understand it. Disenfranchised grief, you may say.

The women's perception of how others viewed their grief significantly impacted those specific relationships and played a huge factor in their loneliness. But most importantly, the women admitted that their pregnancy loss had changed them and their capacity to relate with people around them.

Relationships may break down because of incongruent forms of grief.

This change extended to the women's relationships with their partners. The loss and subsequent trauma and grief change you and your partner. Ultimately, some of the women in the study admitted that their perception of themselves and their partners changed. They had to learn new ways of accommodating the new person after the loss had changed them and the marriage. This makes pregnancy loss even more complicated. You lose a child, hope for the future, the possibility of being a mother, and most importantly, your former self. You lose that familiar way of relating to your loved ones and former way of existence.

A few women in the study thought these changes impacted their lives positively, i.e., they strengthened their relationships with people close to them. However, many women didn't share this opinion. There was a sense of ambiguity around how the loss transformed them and its impact on their relationships. For example, one woman admitted that she felt more envious and was less tolerant of people after her pregnancy loss.

"I was never envious before losing. I was very happy with my life; I never wished for anybody else's life. I was a fairly calm kind of person. But now I think, jeez, I wish that could be me. And I don't cope with stress as much as I used to. I don't tolerate people as much either. I am like, get over it! I am a different person. Not necessarily better, but different."

Many women develop a unique perspective of the world after pregnancy loss. Their perspective of themselves and how they interact with the world shifted. Previous studies show that loss and grief can increase an individual's understanding of their willpower and strength and create stronger bonds between them and their loved ones. Pregnancy loss may bring about an improved sense of compassion, but the resulting personal change may not always be positive.

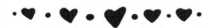

A personal story from a woman shared about being a single woman with pregnancy loss.

Losing a pregnancy is tough enough, but it's different when you go through it alone. It's different when there is no one to share the grief with or even to comfort you. This is every woman's nightmare, but it was the reality of one woman who shared her story and had it published by *The Washington Post.*

Susan Henderson shares that when she first thought of being a mom, she was slightly surprised by this desire. She was almost 40, single, happy, and living her best life. She had a great relationship with her friends and her family. Her family was loving and supportive, and her friends were great. She'd had a fulfilling career, and she loved her job. And the cherry on top was her two beautiful dogs which she doted on. Her life was complete, and she was grateful for it. I mean, what more could someone ask for?

Motherhood was not in her cards. She'd never held a baby, changed a diaper, or babysat before.

But as Susan approached 40, she reflected on her life and decisions. It quickly dawned on her that she might regret not being a mother down the road, and it might be too late. She admits she wasn't interested in speed dating. She didn't want to find some random guy she would drag down the aisle or try a one-night stand and hope for the best. Her respect for marriage and men couldn't let her go down that road. What about adoption? Well, that didn't sit right with her either.

There was only one ethical and safe alternative for her: pregnancy and birth.

She thoroughly researched the best fertility clinics and the available sperm banks and donors. She also prayed a lot during the process. She didn't know what to expect. As she dug deeper into her research, she thought and hoped she would change her mind. To bring around a little one into this world alone and raise them without a father was a difficult thought. She was raised a Christian in a traditional, conservative Southern Baptists household, so this was one of the hardest decisions she was faced with. She didn't think her life would turn out this way.

But after much thought and consideration, Susan realized that this was something she could do. She was confident she could provide her child with a safe and loving home. After all, families are built in different ways. There was a whole village behind her. The child would have loving grandparents, amazing uncles and aunties, and many wonderful friends. Susan knew that even as a single parent, she could provide her child with a beautiful, loving life.

She was confident in her decision because she knew many women who'd had children in their 40s. The fertility numbers for someone her age was above average, according to her doctors and healthcare providers. Still, she didn't have lots of time. With every passing month, the possibility of carrying a pregnancy became riskier and less likely. Studies show that while some women successfully carry a pregnancy to term and deliver a healthy baby in their 40s, many others don't and can't. Susan quickly learned that the rate of miscarriage for women her age was higher, approximately 30%.

Susan was excited and thrilled when she got pregnant quickly through intrauterine insemination. Even more exciting was the great news she learned at the first ultrasound appointment; she was having twins. She fell in love immediately. She listened to those two heartbeats for a long time, and happy tears welled in her eyes. She could also see her twins' tiny fingers moving around. After this, she started shopping in preparation for the twins' arrival. She bought double strollers and matching outfits, picked beautiful twins' names, and thought of how beautiful her life would be. She imagined the beauty and chaos of her life with two dogs, two kids, and a full-time job. Her hands were going to be full.

Sadly, this would never happen.

On May 28th, 2012, at 4 a.m., Susan woke up to severe pain in her abdomen. She was shocked to find herself lying in a pool of blood. Shocked, she dragged herself to the phone and called her clinic's emergency number. They advised her to go to the ER immediately. Susan describes herself as being shocked, too stunned to cry. She held onto her belly and talked to her twins. She was pleading with God, asking Him to let them be okay. She would also speak to the twins, telling them how much she loved them. A close friend wheeled her into the ER as she was still processing everything.

In the ER, the healthcare provider confirmed that there was only one heartbeat. There was still hope for one of her babies, but she had already lost one of them. The remaining twin's heartbeat was strong, and Susan was sent home on bed rest after a few days at the hospital. She was heartbroken but relieved that one of the twins had made it. Three days later, she woke up with the same symptoms she'd had a few days ago. She immediately knew what had happened. A quick trip to the ER confirmed her worst fears. There was no heartbeat anymore. The remaining "products of conception" had to be removed quickly so she wouldn't develop an infection.

Susan broke down. How could this happen to her? She had tried her best to do everything as instructed. She didn't take *alcohol, caffeine, or any food she was told to avoid. She took the right foods and her vitamins as instructed and read multiple books and blogs about having healthy pregnancies. She exercised, but not too much.*

Susan was overwhelmed by her emotions and sadness; the grief consumed her. She blamed herself and asked herself so many questions. Is there something she did that caused the pregnancy loss? Her healthcare provider told her that she hadn't, and it wasn't her fault. The fetal tissue tests and tests on her didn't reveal anything. But Susan was overwhelmed with guilt. Maybe something happened, she wondered. She second-guessed herself. She felt lifeless, like a zombie. A dilation and a curettage were used to remove the remaining blood and tissue after the miscarriage, but the uterus didn't clear up. She described her physical pain as horrific; nothing can be compared to it. She spent many hours on the bathroom floor curled up in a ball, crying herself sick. In every way, her life seemed to split into two parts; before and after the pregnancy loss.

Going through this alone was, in some ways, a blessing and a curse in others. No one else was as invested in the babies as she was. She had no one to cry with in the middle of the night when she was overwhelmed by grief. She had no one to hold on to as she cried or someone to share the loss with as a parent.

On the flip side, she didn't have a family or a marriage to worry about. There was no marriage to nurture or family to maintain, so she was free to focus on her grief and pain at that moment. She didn't have to worry about another person's grief while dealing with her own. For her, this was a relief. Her two greyhounds comforted her when she was most miserable. She reached out to her social networks and shared her story with them. She was blown away by how many had also lost their pregnancies. When her friends and co-workers told her about their experiences with pregnancy loss, she didn't feel as alone or isolated as she had at first.

She also joined other support groups online, and the women there took her under their wing and made her feel better. Susan realized that while pregnancy loss wasn't normal, it was more common than she thought. Her babies were real, and she was saddened that she wouldn't see them grow up and have their own lives, kids, jobs, etc. She then realized there are no ceremonies for these kinds of losses, no flowers, funerals, or church services. She'd suffered one of humanity's biggest and most difficult losses, and only a few people knew.

When she turned 40, Susan decided to try again, but through a different method; in-vitro fertilization (IVF). There is so much that goes into an IVF; belly shots, pills, butt shots, patches, etc. IVF isn't for the faint-hearted, Susan admits. She gained weight, had breakouts, her hair turned grey, and others fell off. She became darker and had bruises all over. Susan miscarried two other pregnancies, most of which happened earlier on in the pregnancies. They all happened at home, where she was all alone.

By this time, she was physically and emotionally exhausted. She quietly cleaned up and made an emergency call to her doctor. She searched for online support groups for women who'd had multiple miscarriages. Slowly, she started accepting that maybe she would never be a mother. She wanted to give up but couldn't bring herself to do it. Her loved ones were worried sick about her physical and mental health. Many of them asked why she didn't stop and kept trying. She didn't know what to tell them except that she couldn't give up.

There was only one egg left at her fertility clinic by late 2014. Susan admits that at this point, she had already given up on her dream of being a mother and started moving on. She decided to try with this last one, telling herself that maybe she would miscarry again, which would be the end of everything for her. Only this time, she didn't lose the pregnancy. This last egg became the survivor. At 30 weeks, she announced her pregnancy to her family and friends on Facebook. She was open about everything she'd gone through and the losses she had to overcome.

At 42, Susan gave birth to her son. She will never get over losing her other kids, but it's a loss she's learned to live with.

Single women may choose this path and can find support and grieve with others.

Single Mothers by Choice is an institution that was established in 1981 to support and empower women who've chosen to have children knowing they'll be their child's sole parents, at least for a start. Jane Mattes founded the organization, and more than 30,000 women have enjoyed its benefits since then. Single Mothers by Choice provides information and support to single mothers throughout the US, Europe, Canada, and beyond.

The organization has local chapters and an online private Discussion Forum active 24/7. They also have newsletters and are more than willing to share their resources, expertise, and experiences with women who want to or are single mothers by choice. The organization provides resources on topics such as Parenting, Thinking, Planning, and Becoming a single mother by choice, available donor options, and insemination, among other things. This is an inclusive organization that doesn't discriminate against anybody. They welcome people from all backgrounds, gender, culture, race, social status, etc.

Single Mothers by Choice is a good organization that provides help and support for all single women who've experienced pregnancy loss. You don't have to be a single mother by choice to access and benefit from their services. Even if you became pregnant unintentionally as a single woman and suffered pregnancy loss, you can find help and support there. If you have no one supporting you in the intense grief and heartache, feel free to contact the organization through their website and be part of the thousands of women they've helped and supported. Find their website in the Resources section of the book.

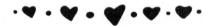

Six

Wholesome Body

♥

Pregnancy loss is deeply felt and can have long-drawn physical, mental, and spiritual impacts on you and the people around you. As the grief changes you, it will also change your relationships with your friends, family, yourself, partner, and other children. Most importantly, your body will experience many changes after a pregnancy loss. It's important to understand and know what to expect after a miscarriage or stillbirth so you and your loved ones can grieve and find healing after the loss. With this knowledge, you'll also know what to look for regarding signs and symptoms that indicate complications or infections and how to give your body that loving care and attention it deserves.

Common physical symptoms after miscarriage and stillbirth

Your symptoms will be determined by the length of the pregnancy you lost.

Here's what to expect depending on when the loss happened:

An early pregnancy loss

- You'll experience menstrual-like bleeding for several days

- Cramping for several days

- Continuous spotting for up to four weeks

Suppose you had a dilation and curettage (D&C)

Dilation or curettage (D&C) is a miscarriage involving any form of medication/medical termination. You can expect:

- Cramping for several days after the termination

- Light bleeding several days after the termination

- Diarrhea

- Nausea

After a stillbirth

- Heavy bleeding that can last up to six weeks

- Abdominal cramps

- Body aches

- Discomfort in the perineal area

- Fatigue

- Postpartum symptoms include bleeding, soreness, difficulty urinating, constipation, hemorrhoids, puffy/bloodshot eyes, sweating at night, sore nipples, and enlarged breasts. Your breasts may leak, and you may struggle with back pain.

Emotions don't have a timeline. They can take you days, weeks, or even months to process. Unlike your body which recovers quickly, your emotional healing may not be so straightforward. You'll cramp and bleed for a few days after an early pregnancy loss. Your menses typically come back after four to six weeks. This is a hint that your body is ready for a new pregnancy if you'd like to try again.

The symptoms accompanying later pregnancy losses are more intense and usually last longer. As heartbreaking as it may sound, the physical symptoms of stillbirth are identical to live birth. You'll experience labor and all the other discomforts associated with live birth. The bleeding may stop after six weeks, and then you'll experience cramping as the uterus shrinks into its original size.

It may take approximately four weeks for all the contents of the uterus to be expelled after a miscarriage. During this time, you'll experience spotting and light bleeding, which are completely normal. Avoid having sexual intercourse during this time. Don't put anything in your vagina either, e.g., tampons. These can cause infections which may complicate issues even further. Your body will go back to the way it was soon.

Dilation and curettage (D&C) is minor surgery to remove tissues left in the uterus after pregnancy loss. This exact procedure is used during elective medical terminations. You may experience mild to moderate cramps after this, and mild painkillers can be prescribed. If general anesthesia was used during the process, you might feel nauseous. You'll feel better after a few days following the surgery. You must avoid sexual intercourse, tampons, or anything put inside the vagina for a few weeks.

When should you call a doctor?

Complications and infections may happen after pregnancy loss. Pay attention to the signs and symptoms. Call a medic or go to the ER if you experience any of the following:

In case of a miscarriage

- Abdominal pains

- Chill or fever

- Smelly discharge

- Bleeding that lasts longer than a week

In the case of a D&C

- Chills or fever

- Intense abdominal pain

- Smelly discharge

- Heavy menses that last longer than your usual period

In case of stillbirth

- Chills or fever

- Severe headaches

- Seizures

- Chest pains

- Swollen legs

- Heavy bleeding or passing clots

- Difficulty breathing

Pregnancy loss is hard. Take all the time necessary to heal and go easy on yourself. Soon enough, your body will recover and restore to some state of normalcy.

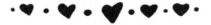

7 Things to do after a miscarriage for self-care

To avoid complications, you must act immediately after a miscarriage, according to expert gynecologists. Miscarriages, just like any other losses, are emotionally and physically overwhelming to a woman's body and spirit. In reality, miscarriages lead to severe mental anguish and physical distress. For this reason, it's imperative to do certain things immediately after a miscarriage for faster recovery of the mind and spirit.

So, what should you do after a miscarriage?

- **You might want to rest for at least a week if the miscarriage happens within the first trimester.**

Rest is essential, even if the pregnancy loss happened earlier in the pregnancy. Stay home and rest as much as necessary. This is the best way to regulate the bleeding that follows a miscarriage.

- **You might need bed rest if the loss happened between the 6th – 8th week**

In this case, you'll need complete bed rest for at least six weeks after the miscarriage. Consume healthy, nutritious foods, particularly those rich in iron, calcium, and vitamins. Healthier food options and rest from regular activities speed up recovery.

- **Stay away from household chores.**

It would help if you didn't pick up anything for now or do any heavy-duty household chores during this time. Household tasks may complicate an already difficult situation by causing discomfort and pain. This is where your partner or loved ones can come in and help. Ask for assistance where necessary.

- **Take your medication regularly.**

Your doctor will prescribe the much-needed medication for your recovery. Take your medicine on time and regularly, without skipping a day. This is the only way to avoid pregnancy loss-related infections. If you are going to therapy, don't skip your appointments, even when you don't feel like going. Keeping up with your appointments and medication is the first step toward physical recovery.

- **You may want to avoid sex for now.**

The uterus is sensitive and delicate as it is. Add the trauma of a miscarriage, and it becomes extremely sensitive, which would explain why gynecologists advise you to avoid sexual intercourse after pregnancy loss. Wait for a while, at least until after the bleeding stops. However, the recommended time is a six-week gap following the loss. Take your time to avoid complications and speed up the recovery process.

- **Don't douche**

I am not sure if I can stress this enough, but douching after a pregnancy loss is an absolute NO! Douching at any time is not necessary for the vagina's natural flora. Moreover, you should avoid any vaginal wash after a miscarriage.

- **Postpone rigorous workout sessions**

Your body has gone through a lot; it needs rest to recover from the physical trauma of the loss. You can pick up your beloved strength training, cardio, high-intensity weight training, and any other intense workouts later, but your health should come first for now. If you must exercise, then yoga, some simple breathing techniques, and light exercise routines should do. Meditation also works and helps keep you calm and stress-free.

Most importantly, stay in touch with your gynecologist after the miscarriage until you fully recover. Be vigilant and check for signs associated with pregnancy loss-related complications such as acute abdominal pain, heavy bleeding, fever, or any unnatural smell from the vagina. Go to the ER as soon as you spot any of these symptoms. You must also under-

stand that life is stressful and overwhelming, and miscarriages happen; it's not your fault or anybody else's.

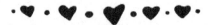

**But what if it was a stillbirth? How do you cope and prac-
tice self-care then?**

Stillbirths are heartbreaking, and this moment may stay with
you as long as you live. You did the hard work of going
through excruciating labor and delivery, and now, you must
think about what follows. You may be curious; how will this
affect my body? What does recovery after a stillbirth look
like? Will I ever learn to process the loss to the point where I
can finally accept it?

Sadly, many of these questions may remain unanswered for
a while. However, I know that if you take time to process the
grief, rest, learn what to expect, and find ways to honor the
loss, your physical and emotional recovery might be just a
little bit easier.

But first, what happens after a stillbirth?

Well, the first few days and weeks following a stillbirth may
feel and seem like a scary, horrific blur. The truth is, no two

experiences after a stillbirth are alike, but the expectation is that your pain will be fresh and raw. You are still in the initial stages of grief and are only learning to process your loss while dealing with the challenging physical experiences of a c-section or a natural or induced labor. You'll be required to go through several tests at some point. An autopsy may be conducted on the baby to determine the real cause of the stillbirth.

Visit your gynecologist regularly after the stillbirth. Your healthcare provider will examine you during these visits to determine your physical progress thus far. The doctor will bring up the autopsy results and the results of your tests. These visits allow you to get your questions answered and understand the potential for trying again if you are interested.

Your recovery after a stillbirth and how long it takes depends, to a great extent, on how the birth happened. Was it a C-section, natural, or induced labor, maybe? But whether the birth was vaginal or a c-section, you can expect your physical and emotional recovery to be conflicting and confusing. Moreover, the shock, numbness, devastation, and hopelessness that follows stillbirth may be so overwhelming that it completely overshadows your physical healing.

Care after vaginal stillbirth

You'll experience postpartum bleeding, medically known as lochia, after the vaginal delivery. Your uterus works all round the clock to get rid of blood, tissue, and mucus left after the loss. The bleeding starts like regular menses and tapers off gradually over time, taking up to six weeks. Expect small clots and heavy bleeding during the process, but get in touch with your healthcare provider if you notice larger clots (clots bigger than grapes) or bleed through a pad per hour.

You may also notice swelling and pain around the perineum (the tissue between your anus and vulva). The pain and swelling may cause discomfort, which may last for a few weeks depending on whether or not some tearing occurred or how long the labor was. Try regular sitz baths to minimize the soreness. You can also ice the area every few hours after the birth; this helps.

As you urinate, the torn skin may sting and burn a little; this is completely normal. Fortunately, the stinging and burning ease up after a while. Spray the area with warm water using a peri bottle before and after your bathroom visit to minimize the discomfort.

Care after a c-section stillbirth

The recovery process following a c-section stillbirth may take longer than vaginal birth. You'll stay a while at the hospital and rest longer when you get home. Your body may only start to recuperate after around four to six weeks following the birth. You will experience many, if not all, symptoms associated with vaginal delivery, including bleeding, cramping, and perineal soreness. You'll also itch, chaff, and experience numbness in the incision area. Pain-relieving drugs will help you manage the pain and discomfort.

Sanitize the incision area regularly to reduce the chances of infection. Call your healthcare provider immediately if there are signs the wound isn't healing properly. Signs to look out for include oozing, pus, redness, or fever.

You were given anesthesia before the c-section; it may slow down your digestion, causing bloating and gassiness. The subsequent bloating and gassiness put pressure on the c-section incision, causing irritation and discomfort. If you can, stay away from gaseous foods at this time. Try lying on your back or left side. While on your back, draw your knees up, take deep breaths, and hold the incision. Doing this may provide some relief.

You may also experience other symptoms, including:

-

Fatigue; remember, you went through labor and delivery just like you would in a live birth.

- Cramping and afterpains. Your uterus must contract back to its original size.

- Swelling around the ankles, feet, and legs. Don't be alarmed when your face swells, too; it's completely normal. Postpartum hormonal shifts, IV fluids, and other factors may cause swelling.

- The hormonal shifts may cause night sweats too. This is how your body regulates and sheds off the extra fluids.

- Breast leaking and swelling are normal too.

- Constipation.

- You may have trouble urinating.

- Hemorrhoids associated with pushing during delivery.

- Back pain and other body aches and pains.

It's possible that because of everything you are going through emotionally, you may neglect your physical recovery. However, it's important to stay in touch with your healthcare provider if you notice any signs of infection mentioned above or the complications mentioned below:

- Very heavy bleeding.

- Red, swollen feet that feel tender when touched.

- Severe headaches that don't go away after treatment.

- Fever – from 100.4 degrees F. or higher.

- When the incision doesn't heal.

- Chest pains.

- Seizures.

- Trouble breathing.

Lactation

The body prepares itself for your baby's arrival during pregnancy and delivery by producing hormones that help it produce milk and colostrum. Your doctor may, in most cases, suggest dopamine agonists that turn off milk and colostrum production after pregnancy loss. The dopamine production also limits breast engorgement and leaking as much as possible. Unfortunately, dopamine agonists can't be given to women with preeclampsia.

It's okay if you'd rather not use medication that stops lactation. The body, at some point, will stop milk production naturally. This may take longer, though, and you may experience more engorgement and leaking. Cold compresses and over the counter pain-relievers, such as ibuprofen, may reduce the discomfort.

What to expect after medical termination - the physical symptoms and emotional recovery

Medical termination of a pregnancy is one of the most difficult decisions anyone will ever have to make. Medical termination of a pregnancy will take a toll on you emotionally; it may not be easy. It's a difficult decision, and as expected, your recovery will differ from other types of pregnancy losses.

What should you expect?

First, the physical recovery will be dependent on the specific type of procedure you had. The termination may be a D and C involving removing all the products of conception, the fetus, and the placenta from the uterus. Based on your physical health and how far along you are in the pregnancy, you may undergo an outpatient surgical procedure or use medication to terminate the pregnancy.

You'll experience pain in either case, followed by bleeding and cramping. Some antibiotics may be prescribed to minimize the risk of infection.

Medical abortions/medication abortions

Your doctor will give you some drugs you are to take while you are still at their office and others that you'll carry home and take 24-48 hours after the first dose. Expect cramping and heavy bleeding after taking the medication. The bleeding and cramping may last for several hours. Pads are recommended, but if you prefer menstrual cups or tampons, check in with your doctor to ensure it's okay.

You may experience other symptoms, including:

- Chills

- Fever

- Nausea

- Vomiting

- Diarrhea

- Light bleeding or spotting may continue for up to two weeks

Avoid physically demanding activities for a few days after the termination. Visit your doctor after the procedure to ensure every product of conception has been cleared up from the uterus. If not, a surgical procedure to clear up everything might be necessary. Expect your regular period four to six weeks after the procedure.

Surgical abortions

The procedure done in the case of surgical abortion is almost identical to dilation and curettage (D&C). A suction-like device is used to dilate and remove all the products of conception.

You may experience:

- Drowsiness

- Cramping for several hours

- Bleeding

- Spotting

- Headaches

- Diarrhea

- Vomiting

Your doctor will prescribe some antibiotics to minimize the risk of infection associated with the procedure. It would help if you rest and avoid rigorous activities during this time until you fully recover. Expect your period four-to-six weeks after the pregnancy.

Cramping after surgical termination of a pregnancy can be managed using over the counter painkillers. It's best, however, to ask your healthcare provider for advice on this. Your doctor may prescribe stronger pain alternatives if the pain is severe. You may want to avoid sexual intercourse; wait until the bleeding stops to minimize the risk of infections and complications.

There's always a risk of infection, whichever method of medical termination you choose. You should, therefore, take your prescribed medication and get in touch with your doctor if you experience any of the following:

- Severe back or abdominal pain that worsens over time

- Heavy bleeding, which would be described as soaking at least two pads in an hour for two hours continuously

- Foul-smelling discharge

- Fever - 100.4 degrees F. or more

Emotional Recovery after Medical Termination

Your emotional recovery will be difficult if your decision is riddled with regret and guilt, even when you know it's the right decision. The termination may have happened early, but you'll still deal with many emotions. It's okay to feel this way.

You may find yourself mourning the loss and feeling guilty about the decision. You made the right call for yourself, your loved ones, and your partner, so don't beat yourself up or put yourself down for something already done. You also have a right to mourn, grieve and feel however you do. You have every right to mourn the best way you see fit and remember the baby the best way you know how. There isn't a right or invalid way to deal with or mourn this type of loss or any other loss.

Rest if you must, and take time to make sense of your thoughts and emotions. Speak up and involve your partner if you have one; it will help and make a massive difference in their journey toward recovery. It's not just you mourning, so share your feelings with and help each other. Join support groups of people who've been through the same. Spiritual advisors, therapists, and grief counselors are excellent re-sources too.

You can create a reflective activity to honor your lost child's memory if you wish. Honoring your child in whichever way can be incredibly healing. Plant a tree, flowers, or a beauti-ful garden. Plan a commemorative meal in their honor and invite your close friends and family, have a simple picnic with your partner, alone, or with a close one, light a candle, observe a few quiet moments, or express your feelings and emotions by writing a heartfelt letter to the baby. Say goodbye in your own way, a way that gives you a sense of peace and closure.

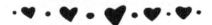

Physical activity after pregnancy loss

Exercise is most likely one of the last things you want to do after a miscarriage or stillbirth. You probably wonder if it's safe to engage in physical activity after pregnancy loss. Well, studies show that physical activity is critical after pregnancy loss, even in milder forms. Exercise will help you recoup your strength in mind, body, and spirit and helps reduce depression, anxiety, and stress following the loss. Physical activity also allows you to "reintegrate back" and adjust to being around others again. It eases muscle tension and improves sleep patterns.

Sadly, physical activity is still under-recommended by healthcare practitioners. Women leave after stillbirth, for example, with a body that still looks pregnant and no baby. Health teaching beyond "return to normal activity" is not given. Why is that? The critical question here is; why are women who've had live births encouraged to exercise, and the benefits of such are evident in literature targeting such women when the same is openly missing in women who've experienced pregnancy loss?

Studies show that women who've experienced pregnancy loss would appreciate physical activity-related advice from their healthcare providers, just like women who've had live births. Still, reports show that up to 61% of women exercised following their stillbirths. This could be because many believe or know that being active helps them feel better. Women who were active during pregnancy maintained these habits following a stillbirth, reportedly admitting that physical activity helped them cope with their new reality, feel better, and have some much-needed alone time.

Light to moderate physical activity gives you an outlet and builds your self-esteem and self-confidence. It's not unusual that many women lose faith in their bodies' abilities after the loss, but many admit that exercise helps them feel stronger. Physical activity has been proven as an effective non-pharmacological method that helps reduce depressive symptoms, anxiety, grief symptoms, and episodic relapses.

Your healthcare provider may recommend lighter, modified versions of the same exercise routine you followed during pregnancy. If you weren't a marathoner, it wouldn't make sense to pick up the habit after pregnancy loss. It's essential to find balance and check in with your doctor before starting any strenuous activity.

Your body will probably return to how it was pretty quickly if the loss happened in the first trimester, which means you can return to your regular exercise routine quickly. Provided your symptoms, including cramping, bleeding, and aches, are being monitored by a doctor, you can resume exercise soon after a second-trimester loss. Unless you've been advised not to, there is no reason why you shouldn't exercise. Most importantly, however, is to listen to your body, take it easy, and move at your own pace. You might feel the need to push yourself, but be gentle with yourself. Let your body take on what it can naturally handle.

Start your physical activity journey with low-impact exercises discussed below:

- **Walking**

This is one of the best forms of physical activity after pregnancy loss. Walking gives you a chance to process complex emotions and move painful experiences through your body. You can also walk with your partner, a close friend, or a family member. They can make it easier on you, and while you are at it, they get a chance to talk more openly about the loss.

Sometimes, getting out of the house alone may seem difficult, impossible even, and this is normal and understandable.

I mean, walking past other pregnant women and others holding their babies may be difficult. Maybe you are worried about how you look – you may still look pregnant; it's okay if you don't want to. When you finally feel like you can, take some short strolls and enjoy the fresh air. Get into nature or any beautiful place that calms the spirit.

- **Yoga**

Stretching exercises give you flexibility and help you tone your body, and they aren't too strenuous. You can dim your light, light some candles, and put on some soothing music as you engage in gentle or restorative yoga. Yoga helps calm and relax your mind and spirit.

- **Water aerobics**

You don't have to do too much or try too hard, but being afloat helps take away the pressure off your joints and body. It's okay if you don't feel like moving; just start by floating and move along slowly when ready.

- **Pelvic floor exercises**

Your hormones will have affected your pelvic floor, even if the loss happened early in the pregnancy. For this reason, pelvic floor exercises are recommended, but you must only do them when you are strong enough. A stronger pelvic floor protects you from leaking urine and helps with vaginal healing. Pelvic floor exercises improve blood circulation to the area, which helps reduce swelling and bruising. Don't worry about stitches; pelvic floor exercises pose no risk to them at all.

You may feel like your pelvic floor muscles aren't responding in the first few weeks or days, but you must keep going because it works, even if you aren't feeling it yet.

- **Lower tummy muscle exercises**

Working out your lower tummy area helps you reduce the post-pregnancy belly. These muscles and lower pelvic muscles help support your pelvis and back.

- **Pelvic tilts**

Pelvic tilts are important after pregnancy loss. They help move and stretch the back area and tummy muscles. This way, the pelvic tilts help with back pain also. Try doing them while sitting, lying down, or with an exercise ball.

If you are still worried about your physical abilities after pregnancy loss, bring a loved one or work with a trainer to help monitor your progress as you exercise.

Foods to eat for healing and foods to avoid

Pregnancy loss is hard on the body, and it may take a while to bounce back to everyday life. The most important thing, however, is to take care of your physical and mental health. Food is medicine and it's how we fuel and support healing in the body. Here are important dietary factors to keep in mind during this time:

First, while it's essential to follow a nutritious diet to build your energy and stamina back, you don't have to starve from or completely avoid comfort foods when you feel sad or low. Above all, eat a healthy diet that provides you with essential nutrients. Nutrition helps you manage the weakness, weight loss, and bleeding associated with pregnancy loss.

Do Eat:

- **Foods rich in proteins**

Your body makes use of the amino acids found in proteins to build new tissue and replace damaged cells. Protein-rich foods help speed up your recovery and healing process.

Foods rich in proteins include – fish, meat, eggs, milk, lentils, grains, cheese, quinoa, etc.

- **Folate-rich foods**

Many healthcare providers recommend folate-rich foods for health during and after pregnancy. Folate quickens the recovery process after pregnancy loss. They include leafy green vegetables, including spinach, kales, lettuce, seeds, and nuts.

- **Foods rich in calcium and magnesium**

Magnesium deficiency increases the risk of depression, according to multiple studies. Eating magnesium and calcium-rich foods reduces pregnancy loss-related stress, anxiety, and depression. Again, leafy green vegetables are rich in magnesium. Eat more whole grains such as brown rice, oatmeal, and barley. Dairy products also provide your body with the calcium it needs after pregnancy loss. You can always supplement with Vitamin C and magnesium found in any health store.

- **Foods rich in iron and vitamins**

Iron and vitamin-rich foods quicken recovery and improve your body's iron absorption capabilities. These foods also help with other symptoms, including weakness and blood loss. Dates, raisins, oranges, fish, and beans are excellent sources of iron and vitamins.

- **Take plenty of fluids.**

Bleeding and blood loss are synonymous with pregnancy loss. Therefore take plenty of fluids to replace the lost fluids. Try coconut water and other detox drinks to improve absorption. Turmeric milk before sleeping also helps. Pomegranate juice can also help maintain the correct body fluid levels.

Avoid:

- **Sodas**

Multiple studies report that taking sodas regularly affects fertility. Sodas have high levels of caffeine that add nothing to the recovery or healing process. Stay away from artificial sweeteners, too; they raise blood sugar levels and slow recovery.

- **Alcohol**

Abstain from alcohol after pregnancy loss. Not only after pregnancy loss, but alcohol isn't great for your health, especially in large volumes or frequency. Talk to your doctor about the best alcohol-quitting methods.

- **Processed Food**

Burgers, pizzas, fries, etc., should be avoided after a mis-carriage. Junk foods provide empty calories that raise blood sugar and do nothing regarding healthy nutrients. They fill your stomach for a while, but it is all in vain because they contribute nothing to your recovery.

- **Sugary foods**

Sugary foods like sweets, chocolate, cakes, etc., fall in the same class as junk. Stay away from them after the pregnancy loss. Sugary foods raise your blood sugar levels and may give rise to other problems. The sugar fluctuations in the blood-stream may also interfere with the healing process. Replace unhealthy sugary foods with healthier fruits and vegetables rich in natural sugars.

- **Soy products**

Soy foods are generally nutritious, but they aren't recom-mended after pregnancy loss. They contain the compound phytate, which inhibits iron absorption. Good examples of soy products include tempeh, soybeans and milk, and tofu.

Natural remedies

- **Rest**

As I mentioned, rest is essential after pregnancy loss. Your doctor will advise on how much rest is necessary following the type of pregnancy loss and what stage of pregnancy you were in. You'll need help with regular household chores and childcare. This way, you'll have enough time to relax and recover. Listen to your body.

- **Herbs**

Herbs can play an important role in your recovery process. Use yarrow for blood loss and cramp bark for cramping. Red raspberry leaf tea helps nourish and tone your uterus, minimizes blood loss, and helps you maintain healthy iron levels. Motherwort slows bleeding and improves your mood. Herbs like ashwagandha also help ease pain from cramping and balance your hormone levels.

- **Nourishing foods**

Healthy fruits, vegetables, and plenty of drinks improve hydration and fasten the healing process. Comfort foods like dark chocolate, coconut milk, and chickpeas can also help. Avoid inflammatory foods, including sugary drinks and alcohol.

- **Hot compresses**

Cramping is common and normal after pregnancy loss. Use hot compresses around your back, lower abdomen, and head to reduce pains and aches.

- **Baths**

One important thing to think about after a miscarriage is good hygiene. Proper hygiene reduces the risk of infection and excessive blood loss. Yoni steams and herb baths are good self-care strategies during this period. Try sea salts on your baths and steams too. You can add herbs like sage, garlic, lavender, rosemary, and shepherds' purse to your baths.

- **Abstain for a while**

To prevent infection, avoid sexual intercourse until bleeding stops.

- **Monitor yourself**

Infection and excessive blood loss are two main medical concerns following pregnancy loss. Monitor your symptoms the best way possible at home. Don't skip your appointments, and get your iron levels checked regularly. Studies show that anemic women are more prone to depression, anxiety, and infections.

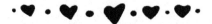

Seven

Mindfulness and Holistic Methods to Reduce Stress

♥

D epression and anxiety are closely related. For a long time, psychologists thought mental health disorders were like fish ponds, where the person suffering was completely isolated in a watertight section. This couldn't be further from the truth. New studies show that these ponds don't exist; there isn't distinct isolation of the different types of mental health disorders. Many are combined, with some displaying some or all of their unique characteristics in a way that affects or exacerbates the "existing" illness.

Psychologists believe that there is a good likelihood that an existing mental health condition favors the occurrence of another over time. Simply, multiple mental health disorders may develop from unrelated causes. An excellent example of this scenario is depression and anxiety. These two mental health disorders are distinct and many cases of people suffering from them separately exist. Still, there is always a strong chance that they'll appear combined in what experts call mixed anxiety-depressive disorder (MADD).

The existence of MADD rings true after perinatal loss and in women who are pregnant again following prior pregnancy loss. Indeed, depression and anxiety are distinct and can be suffered separately, but they are not entirely exclusive. Both anxiety and depression have high adverse effects resulting from severe emotional pain. They are both characterized by deep feelings of sadness, guilt, regret, low mood, internal suffering, irritability, and susceptibility.

Both mental health disorders present deep-seated feelings of helplessness, low self-esteem, and self-confidence. This is the reality of most women who've experienced pregnancy loss. Many feel like they are unable to face their circumstances, they are overwhelmed by their difficulties, and their minds are flooded with feelings of doubt and denial.

In mixed anxiety-depressive disorder, none of the two mental health disorders have prominence over the other. For this reason, the MADD doesn't present as a pure case of anxiety, nor is it as severe as full-blown depression. Still, this combination is strong enough to affect a person intensely. When you suffer from this mixed disorder, you may struggle with extreme worry, periods of low energy alternating with hyperactivation, intrusive thoughts, tremors, panic attacks, low mood, anhedonia (inability to experience pleasure), and tachycardia (fast heart rate over 120 at resting).

Studies show that women who've experienced pregnancy loss are four times more likely to suffer from depressive symptoms than those who had live births. The same survey further reveals women who've experienced prenatal loss are seven times more likely to suffer from PTSD. These findings are shocking and alarming. The powerful impact of pregnancy loss and the subsequent stress affects women deeply.

Over the years, women who've experienced pregnancy loss have been encouraged to find alternative holistic methods for coping with depression, grief, anxiety, and stress. These holistic alternatives may facilitate normal grief so women and their partners can find closure. Mental health disorders can make you feel helpless. The truth is, you are not! There is so much you can do to cope with your new reality. As a holistic coach, nurse, and yogi, I have just brushed the surface of holistic stress reduction techniques.

Try:

Journaling to the unborn child to express grief and journaling for yourself

Journaling is an empowering and accessible technique. It is deeply healing. Journaling gives you an outlet and an opportunity to express yourself without judgment. Write about everything you feel, your anger, grief, guilt, sadness, confusion, and resentment. Write about your hopes for the future, the new reality, and the realization that they'll never happen, at least not for this child. Write to your child like you would talk to a friend sitting right next to you.

Journaling provides an adored piece of memorabilia you can revisit whenever you want. To support you with journaling and your healing journey, there is a companion guide to this book titled "*A Path To Wholeness: Journal Prompts and Affirmations for Coping with Pregnancy Loss.*" It can help guide you of where and how to start journaling. You can buy it on Amazon.

Visualizations and imagining lovingly for the lost child and imagining lovingly for yourself

There was a chance they would have been here to laugh, grow, play and be with you. They could have had birthdays, graduated from school, and had their friends, family, and grandchildren. It stings to think of how life would have been with them in it, but it is also healing to visualize and think about them lovingly. It can be therapeutic in many ways to think of your baby surrounded by love and not just in sadness and grief. Imagine their soul is at peace. Whatever your spiritual or religious beliefs are, the one truth we know is we all pass on from this realm just on different timelines. While this baby's time was unjustly short, you can imagine that your baby is resting and peaceful. Let your imagination play with how that may look, see, smell, and feel.

Imagine lovingly for yourself. How do you want your day ahead to feel? What are your hopes and dreams? What do you desire today? What do you desire in the future? Maybe it is healing or to feel better. Imagine and see yourself out of this dark time, feeling whole, confident, supported, hopeful. How does that look? What are you wearing? Who are you with? What is that conversation you're having? What do you hear? Spend time in these imaginal states every day.

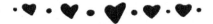

Yoga as an alternative

People continue to practice yoga because of its numerous physical and psychological benefits. Creating a personal yoga routine can help prevent and reduce stress, promote positive change, and focus on understanding and knowing yourself better. You see, yoga is frequently mistaken for being sole poses or asanas. However, in addition to these, a yoga program includes breathing exercises, meditation, and relaxation methods such as yoga Nidra.

Let's look at how yoga can help you cope with depression, anxiety, and stress following child loss:

Clearing your mind

Thoughts don't stop. They are always moving and we have thousands of thoughts in the blink of an eye. Your mind will constantly jump from one thought to the next after losing your child, conjuring up scenarios for the future and replaying unpleasant events from the past. This mental effort is exhausting and stressful. Yoga and meditation practice provides numerous methods for quieting a wandering mind and becoming an observer. As we mentioned earlier, one is breath work. Every breath you take is intimately connected to the present moment; you're not breathing in your past or future. Concentrating only on each inhalation and exhalation puts the focus there on your breath, relieving your focus on any other ideas, clearing your mind, and alleviating stress.

Exercise

Yoga is diverse; some styles are slow and leisurely and more focused on restoration, while others are swift, leaning more toward vigorous exercise and powerful movement. No yoga style is better than another for reducing stress, so choose one that fits your personality and taste as well as level of physical condition.

By keeping your body healthy and generating endorphins, the feel-good hormones, exercise of any kind can help reduce stress. Yoga's stretching techniques also relieve tension.

Relaxation

Savasana, or corpse posture, is one of the most challenging poses with the goal of deeply relaxing which is difficult for many with an active mind. This intended relaxation, though initially challenging, eventually leads to a complete release of the body and mind. It also leaves you feeling rejuvenated and helps you manage stress. In addition, yoga Nidra provides a chance for a more extended, profound period of relaxation. It's also an introduction to meditation, which may be a fantastic stress reliever.

Breath control

Pranayama, often known as breath work, is a crucial component of all yoga practices and carries over well into daily life. At the very least, yoga heightens your awareness of your breath as a means of physical and mental relaxation. Breathing is a necessary and involuntary act for survival but you can control it. Learn the simple art of taking deep breaths when feeling overwhelmed and understand that doing so can help you quickly deal with stressful situations.

Relaxation stress-reduction techniques

Most people think relaxation is lazing out on the couch after a demanding day. This isn't true. Relaxation is an excellent stress reliever. You can achieve relaxation by engaging in the exercises discussed above. Let's look at how you can practice these techniques:

Technique 1: Deep breathing

Deep breathing is a simple yet effective relaxation technique that reduces your stress levels. It's simple to learn, and you can practice it anywhere. To practice this technique, follow the steps below:

- Sit straight-backed in a chair that is comfortable enough with your feet flat on the floor, legs un-crossed. Alternatively, you can sit cross legged on the floor supported by a pillow under your bum.

- Put one hand on your stomach and the other on your chest.

- Take a deep breath through your nose. Your stomach will push out as you fill your belly with breath first and then slowly fill up your lungs to the very top. Your hand will move out. The hand on the chest should only move slightly.

- Breathe through your mouth, forcing out as much air as possible. The hand on the abdomen should move in, but the one on your chest should only move slightly.

- Repeat this process for at least 3 - 10 breaths.

Try lying on your back if you find it challenging to practice this technique while sitting. Put a tiny book on your tummy and breathe such that it rises and falls with each inhalation and exhalation.

Technique 2: Progressive muscle relaxation

This two-step technique involves sequentially tensing and relaxing various bodily muscle groups. Regular practice lets you know intimately how different sections of your body feel under strain and when they are completely relaxed. This helps you respond to the first indications of stress-related physical tension. Consequently, your mind will unwind as your body does.

Here's how to perform this technique:

- Get comfy by wearing loose clothes and taking off your shoes.

- Spend a few moments breathing deeply and steadily.

- Turn your focus to your right foot when you're prepared to do so. Spend a moment concentrating on the sensation.

- Squeeze your right foot's muscles as firmly as you

can. Hold for ten counts.

- Relax your foot. Pay attention to how the foot feels as it becomes loose.

- For a moment, remain in this relaxed condition while taking slow, deep breaths.

- Turn your focus to your left foot. Maintain the same pattern of tension and relaxation in your muscles.

- Contract and relax the various muscle groups as you slowly move up your body.

Try as much as possible to tense the intended muscles only.

Technique 3: Visualization

In visualization, also known as guided imagery, you imagine a peaceful setting where you are free to let go of any tension and anxiety. This is one style of meditation. Pick a location that makes you feel at ease, whether it's a tropical beach, a place you loved as a youngster, or a peaceful forested glen. You can decide to execute your visualization in silence or use hearing aids, such as soothing music, sound machines, or a preferred recording that corresponds to your selected location, like waves on a beach or wind blowing.

To practice visualization, do the following:

Imagine everything in as much detail as possible, including everything you hear, taste, smell, and feel. It's not sufficient to simply "look" at it in your mind's eye like you would a picture. The most satisfactory visualization results come from as many sensory elements as you can imagine.

For instance, suppose you're thinking about a dock on a serene lake:

- See how the sun sets over the sea.

- Listen to the bird song.

- Smell the clean air and pine trees.

- Feel the breeze on your skin.

As you leisurely explore your peaceful location, savor the sensation of your stress fading away. Open your eyes slowly when you're ready and focus on the moment.

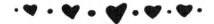

The alternatives

Some people may find it hard to practice the techniques we've discussed above. That's understandable because we're all different. The best part is that there are alternatives you can try that will help you achieve the same results:

Pilates

It's frequently referred to as "yoga's more athletic cousin," even though it's not technically a type of mind-body exercise. Pilates primarily focuses on improving the relationship between the mind and body and reducing stress and tension by fusing your breath with many physical movements. In many aspects, it's pretty similar to several yoga poses ranging from intermediate to advanced. Consequently, you can anticipate a low impact full-body workout that isn't very demanding or strenuous.

Gyrotonics

This workout regimen is arguably similar to yoga because it incorporates elements and motions from tai chi, yoga, gymnastics, swimming, and dance. It's frequently referred to as a brand-new mind-body workout specializing in the body's spirals and arcs.

Gyrotonics works by stretching and strengthening your body. This improves your overall form and posture, enhances your range of motion, and builds physiological co-ordination. It also widens energy channels throughout the body, increases movement effectiveness, and jolts the neurological system.

Dance

It's undeniable that dancing is a fantastic method to express yourself in a variety of diverse physical moves. You might want to experiment with various dance forms if yoga is not your thing. There are many different sorts and styles of dancing to select from, but contemporary dance is the most exciting and spectacular one.

Extreme flexibility, the versatility of movement, physical fitness, complete relaxation, and a way of self-expression are a few major advantages to mental and physical health that contemporary or modern dance offers. This type of dance allows for a certain amount of freedom of movement, allowing the body to pick up on the dance motions with flexibility and incredible ease.

Dance can also be done in a sensual and somatic way where you allow yourself time privately to free flow and get in touch with your body. In my own experience, this style of free dance has been liberating and healing and I use it in my own practice and with coaching clients.

Shaking your body is also a form of somatic therapy where you release trauma from the body by letting go of muscle tension and regulating the nervous system. If you're new to "shaking" start with 10-30 seconds and simply shake out one part of your body. You could be sitting or standing. As you feel more comfortable, progress through other body parts and increase the time of shaking.

Martial arts

Contrary to popular belief, martial arts can be taught and mastered in low-impact environments to improve breathing, physical movement, and balance. They're also not solely for people who want to study the skill of self-defense.

Martial arts have several advantages for both physical and mental health. With this type of physical activity, you should anticipate major increases in your muscles' strength and total cardiovascular fitness.

Tai Chi

This non-competitive martial art mixes easy, gentle physical activities with some stretching and mindfulness techniques. Your body's flexibility, balance, and control are all considerably improved, as is your general fitness. Numerous research on the advantages of Tai Chi for the mind and body has demonstrated that it improves general wellness and health, greatly increases physical strength, relieves chronic pain, and significantly increases fitness and flexibility.

This certainly, by no means, is an exhaustive list of strategies to reduce stress. This is to hopefully inspire you to explore what works for you. If you desire further support with more techniques to calm your mind, reduce anxiety, and feel empowered, go to www.heatheronhealth.com/quietyourmind for a free 5-part video series that I created.

Eight

Releasing Shame and Moving Forward

M any women experience shame and guilt after pregnancy loss because they believe their babies died because they were or aren't "good enough" to be mothers. This false belief of not being enough is one that is universally felt by humans, and exacerbated in times of devastating loss. These feelings can also present as embarrassment over their acts or inactions throughout the pregnancy, especially regarding the experience itself. Because of this, many women frequently keep facts about what occurred a secret, out of concern that it will make them look bad in other people's eyes.

Pregnancy as a "rite of passage"

Your journey to become a parent may be your first Rite of Passage. Every parent's path is different; your pregnancy may be eagerly anticipated or unanticipated, or it may be a joyful surprise. You might be single out of choice or necessity, or you might be in a committed relationship. Your family may or may not be "conventional." You might be thinking about being a supportive partner and a mother. As the pregnancy continues, everyone, especially friends and family members, looks forward to meeting the new family member.

This shows how complex and unique pregnancy is; it's simultaneously social, psychological, biophysical, and developmental. Every pregnancy experience, both good and bad, stays with the mother. With each pregnancy, a mother is in a distinct "life space" as life moves on and relationships develop. A mother forms a unique emotional bond with each child even if the child doesn't survive.

This bond is known as the maternal identity. And when things go contrary to what was anticipated, the mother bears the shame. Breaking the taboo and discussing your loss, therefore, requires courage. Unfortunately, there is so much societal stigma and personal guilt associated with what happens so frequently that it is typically kept a secret. Because child loss is so closely linked to a mother's sense of identity and self-worth, the psychological impacts are severe. There is the sense of being damaged, coupled with excruciating shame. There is the loss of not only the pregnancy but also of your future aspirations for that child.

The lack of discussion of miscarriage in our media and regular conversations heightens its social stigma. In so many ways, it confirms people's perceptions that it's something to be embarrassed about and shouldn't be discussed with others. This is unfortunate because social support is crucial for people dealing with grief following trauma. Consequently, societal stigma stands in the way of a woman who has experienced pregnancy loss, learning that many people out there may have gone through the same thing. It prevents her from recognizing that she's not alone in the experience. If people talked about these issues, many women would understand that they haven't failed as mothers but have experienced a fairly common pregnancy outcome.

Exploring shame

Shame is a common and dominant emotion many of us experience daily. Sadly, shame is typically taboo in modern communities, making it invisible. An analysis of studies on shame shows a taboo that leads to denial and silence. When someone feels humiliated, they strive to cover up their shame. Chronic shame might include the conviction that you're essentially flawed. Shame leads to self-judgment, which becomes problematic when it is internalized. The internal self-critical voice may accuse you of being a bad person, useless, or lacking in value. The truth is, how much shame you experience or feel has little to do with your value or what you've done wrong.

Here are some types of shame:

- **Transient shame** - Transient shame is the momentary emotion you experience after making a mistake, perhaps in front of others. It typically disappears fast and has no negative effects on your life.

- **Chronic shame** - Chronic shame is a feeling that constantly makes you feel unworthy. This type of shame is harmful to your mental and physical health.

- **Shame about defeat** - This kind of shame may strike you in the wake of a setback or loss. For instance, like in losing a pregnancy you were looking forward to.

- **Shame around strangers** - Shame in front of strangers is a sign that you are afraid people will notice you have a problem; that you are imperfect (no one is perfect, though). This type of shame is synonymous with social anxiety.

- **Healthy shame** - It's possible to have healthy shame. It can be beneficial when shame makes you modest, enables you to laugh at yourself, educates you about boundaries, or makes you humble. People wouldn't be able to control how their actions influence others without at least a small amount of shame.

- **Shame from disappointment or failure** - You could experience shame associated with disappointment or failure if you don't meet your goals or if it's taking too long to reach them.

- **Toxic shame** is the idea that something is fundamentally wrong with you. Rather than being a passing feeling, toxic shame is a fundamental component of who you are. Toxic shame sufferers might strive to put on a beautiful exterior to mask how they feel on the inside.

Understanding your shame is the first step to getting over it. This is because if you haven't recognized your shame for what it is, you may not recover from it. To prevent shame from controlling your life, it's important to gain perspective on it, understand its source and how it affects your present decisions. You also need to accept your shame. Although it seems paradoxical, it's essential to bring your internal feelings of guilt into the open if you want to heal from them.

Effects of shame

For some women, shame can be a powerful emotion accompanied by remorse, a sense of failure, and a sense of not being worthy. A surge of post-child loss hormones can cause a storm of confusing feelings, making you feel unlike your "regular" self and giving you the impression that you're going "crazy." Additionally, if you're a person who strives for perfection, feeling as though your body failed you can be a double blow, plunging you further into shame.

Guilt and shame make you feel horrible about yourself, and they sometimes feel incredibly similar. However, guilt might be seen as dissatisfaction with yourself for going against a fundamental internal principle or rule of conduct. Shame, on the contrary, is highly detrimental since it lowers self-esteem and leads to actions that support that negative self-perception.

Shame can be crippling. It causes a variety of issues, including but not limited to:

- Self-criticism and self-blame

- Self-neglect

- Perfectionism

- Self-destructive behaviors

- Self-sabotage

- The conviction that you are not deserving of good things

- Intense rage

- Acting in an unsocial manner

The most effective action you can take to eliminate crippling shame is self-empathy, compassion, and forgiveness. You must learn to forgive yourself if you want emotional health and mental peace.

Practicing self-forgiveness

Self-forgiveness is challenging since it necessitates identifying disturbing emotions and thoughts. Some see the act as a reminder that they are imperfect. Others view it as a strategy for loving yourself despite your flaws. Both are hard, but what would you rather have? If you don't figure out how to embrace self-forgiveness, you may never find internal peace.

Practicing self-forgiveness doesn't mean that you're weak. It does not imply that you are not responsible for what occurred. Furthermore, it doesn't mean that you approved of the events. Self-forgiveness means accepting the events and choosing to move on despite your grief and sadness. Self-forgiveness is good for your relationships and advantageous for your physical and emotional wellbeing.

To effectively practice self-forgiveness, consider the 4 Rs:

Responsibility

The first step toward forgiving yourself is to face the situation, in this case, your pregnancy loss. This is the most challenging step. You may not know the reason why you lost your baby. There is probably no one to blame for this. Regardless of knowing the reason for the loss, there is likely some level of subconscious shame and guilt. The truth of the matter is it happened to you. Accept that this loss is yours, no one else's. It's not your fault and it may not be anyone else's fault either. You are responsible for your own healing after the loss.

Expressing remorse

You may experience difficult emotions, such as guilt and humiliation. It's more beneficial to let these thoughts and feelings out in some way. Keeping them repressed will only exacerbate the pain. Talk about your remorse with a supportive partner, friend, or family member. Discuss these feelings with a therapist, counselor or coach, if you have limited support. Find an outlet either in journaling or voice recording a note. Understand that experiencing this loss feels horrible, but it neither makes you a bad person nor diminishes your inherent worth.

Repairing the damage and restoring the trust

Apologizing is a crucial component of self-forgiveness. Apologize to yourself. Apologize to your baby. It doesn't have to make rational sense. When you apologize, you find freedom from guilt and peace of mind knowing you did your best.

A prayer I practice for forgiveness is the Hawaiian Ho'oponopono prayer.

I'm sorry. Please forgive me. Thank you. I love you.

You may say out loud or silently to your baby, holding your baby in your imagination.

You may say this to yourself.

You may say this to anyone else in your life, past or present, where there needs to be some healing. You don't have to actually say the words to another person. You only need to hold the other person that wronged you in your imagination and repeat this mantra.

Focusing on renewal

Everyone will experience loss and grief at some point in their lives. If you are caught up in self-loathing, self-hatred, or victim mentality about your pregnancy loss, maintaining your self-esteem and motivation is hard. Find a way to learn from difficult trials and challenges and grow from them. To accomplish this, you must first reflect on your actions and your feelings to understand them.

Honoring your lost baby

Due to the possibility of a pregnancy loss, our culture has numerous unspoken guidelines and expectations on how to announce a pregnancy. We believe we are protecting our hearts if we conceal the pregnancy. Our unspoken sadness when we lose the pregnancy may be even more severe. Honoring the life of your deceased child and reflecting on your pregnancy loss can lead to healing.

Here are some creative ways to honor your child:

- **Tattoo**

A tattoo is a terrific expression of your love for your lost child because it's permanent. This will give you a lovely memento of your child. You can consider a short phrase such as "mommy loves you" or "mommy misses you." Baby feet, names, dates, or quotes are all possible tattoo ideas. Because this is something you'll have forever, be careful about the artist you pick and ensure they are skilled enough to do the right thing.

- **Jewelry**

Many lovely jewelry options are available to remind you of your lost child. Birthstone pendants, rings, or an inscribed piece of jewelry are the way to go for more understated jewelry. Additionally, there are numerous memorial jewelry possibilities. For instance, you can search for a local jewelry designer or simply search for "miscarriage jewelry" on Amazon or other big online marketplaces.

- **Planting a tree**

Many moms find great comfort in giving their homes new life. An excellent method to achieve this is planting a tree or flowers. You can bury ashes, the placenta, or other objects underneath the tree.

- **Creating a garden shrine**

This takes it a step further than what we've mentioned above. Establish a peaceful retreat where you can unwind and visit your child. Get a statue or plant flowers that make you think of your child. You can also hang harmony bells on flowers.

- **Teddy bears**

Most organizations make personalized teddy bears the same weight as stillborn children. Holding the teddy bear "child" may give you some comfort.

- **Dedicating a star**

A fantastic alternative is to dedicate a star to your child. It will always be high above, shining down on you, no matter where you go.

- **Write**

Writing has a lot of therapeutic potential. Try journaling or composing a poem to express your emotions. Speak with your child, your family, and yourself. Write whatever you feel helps you heal. For more journaling support, find the companion guide "A Path to Wholeness: Journal Prompts and Affirmations for Coping with Pregnancy Loss" on Amazon.

- **Charity**

Indeed charities aren't a viable option for everyone, but there are times when doing good deeds for others might help in our emotional healing. Consider donating your breast milk through a milk bank to formula-intolerant infants. Other kind acts, including volunteering time at a church or a nursing home, can also be therapeutic.

You can honor your child in various ways. There's no wrong or right way; it's a deeply personal decision only you and your family can make.

The healing journey and triggers

You may recall specific smells, sounds, or pictures associated with the loss of your child. When you come across these sensory recollections, referred to as "triggers," you could experience new feelings of worry, uneasiness, or panic. These triggers accompany the healing process following the loss of your pregnancy. This is completely normal because such emotions don't just go away overnight.

Nowadays, the word "triggered" is used less formally, which may lead to some misunderstandings. But it's crucial to understand that there is a distinction between feeling uneasy or insulted and experiencing a mental health symptom.

Generally, the term "trigger" refers to a stimulus that wakes or exacerbates the symptoms of a traumatic event (child loss) or mental health condition in a person. Others may be surprised by a person's strong response when triggered since the response looks out of proportion to the stimuli. However, this is because the person being triggered is psychologically experiencing the initial trauma.

Our brains tend to retain the surrounding sensory inputs in memory after pregnancy loss. Years later, when we still encounter these sensory cues, the brain may bring back the trauma-related emotions. In certain circumstances, we might not even be aware of the reasons behind our fear or anger. For instance, if the pregnancy loss happens while listening to a particular song or chewing certain bubble gum, they may become triggers when you reencounter them.

However, mental trauma affects each person differently. One scenario may elicit two distinct responses from two people. The other person may acquire PTSD while the other person may come to terms with the traumatic event.

There are many potential causes for this variation in reaction, including the following:

- Personality features and sociocultural background of an individual

- Specific elements of the occurrence

- The significance of the event to the person

Because there is a strong chance you'll encounter specific triggers after pregnancy loss, there are a couple of things you can do to cope with them when it happens:

- **Practice self-acceptance and compassion** - Try not to be angry with yourself for feeling this way. Think of yourself as someone you love and care for, and treat yourself with the same compassion.

- **Consider meditation** - You could also use meditation as a strategy to manage your anxiety. Depression, stress, and anxiety can all be effectively reduced by mindfulness meditation.

- **Keep assuring yourself that you're safe** - Try deep, steady breathing and reassure yourself. Also, you can repeat a mantra that works for you. There were many affirmations shared in the companion guide *"A Path to Wholeness: Journal Prompts and Affirmations for Coping with Pregnancy Loss."*

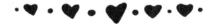

Having another baby

It hurts a lot to experience pregnancy loss. Couples might not want to wait too long to try again after the loss, even when it's evident that recovery takes time. Contrary to popular thinking and even many government guidelines, there is a good possibility that pregnancy following a child loss will succeed. So how soon can you become pregnant after a pregnancy loss?

According to National Institutes of Health Research, women who became pregnant soon after a miscarriage had a more significant live birth percentage (53%) than those who waited longer (36%). In addition, women who become pregnant again within three months of pregnancy loss have a lower risk of miscarriage or stillbirth than those who get pregnant after that time.

This way of thinking is in opposition to advice from very powerful organizations. According to the World Health Organization, couples should wait up to six months following pregnancy loss before trying again. Most of this justification is psychological. Extreme emotional turmoil is unhealthy for pregnant women and their unborn children. Moreover, a higher risk of stillbirth has been associated with grief during pregnancy. Also, depression during pregnancy is linked to a higher risk of mental health issues for the unborn child. But not every person's experience with pregnancy loss is marked by great emotional distress.

So, how soon can you get pregnant following a pregnancy loss? We take into account various limitations to this data because every pregnancy and pregnancy loss is unique. Consult a doctor if the pregnancy loss required any type of medical assistance. This will determine whether to delay getting pregnant again to prevent complications and infections. There are warnings about trying sooner rather than later for couples who have experienced recurrent pregnancy loss or had a miscarriage beyond 13 weeks. Discussing these issues with medical professionals is crucial because they can cause a health risk to the expectant mother and their unborn child.

Even so, the American College of Obstetricians and Gynecologists (ACOG) asserts that there is typically no need to delay the attempt to conceive. Ovulation doesn't start up again until two weeks following a miscarriage. Additionally, waiting two weeks after a loss is advisable before having sex. Most couples might try having a baby at that time. In that case, there might be an advantage to trying immediately. After a miscarriage, fertility may be higher than usual during the first few weeks or months following a pregnancy loss.

Subsequent pregnancies and anxiety

The worry of losing another pregnancy is among the scariest aspects of trying to conceive again. The problem with experiencing a pregnancy loss is that you always worry about it happening again. Early pregnancy loss is so taxing and discouraging that some decide against trying again. That's still okay. The doctor can assess your risk of experiencing another miscarriage based on several variables. There are no absolute certainties, but you might be pleasantly surprised to learn that your likelihood of a safe pregnancy is still high.

Because unpredictable, uncontrollable factors typically bring on pregnancy loss, the worry can grow to epic dimensions. Miscarriage is, unfortunately, a regular occurrence, especially in the first twelve weeks. Even though it's a potential outcome, it shouldn't be your main priority. If you've experienced a pregnancy loss, the likelihood of visiting the doctor more frequently is likewise higher. Blood tests performed more regularly to monitor the baby's health may help you feel better and at peace. It can be comforting to hear a heartbeat during an ultrasound.

While it makes sense to fear another pregnancy loss, the most crucial thing to remember is that the cause of pregnancy loss is frequently unclear. When it happens, neither you nor anybody else is to blame. Losing a pregnancy is neither your fault nor the responsibility of anyone else. You might also want to avoid specific triggers that can worsen your fear and anxiety. For instance, you might wish to see a different OB/GYN when you become pregnant again. Always be honest with those in your support system, even if they're just your partner and your parents.

Here are several ways to combat this fear:

- **Accept that some situations are beyond your control** – Most pregnancy losses are natural and are nobody's fault. Blaming yourself only leads to low self-esteem, guilt, and shame.

- **Don't embrace everything you read online** - Searching for pregnancy loss information online when you are already dealing with fear and anxiety makes you lean more toward the negative information.

- **Focus on what you can do** - Prolonged anxiety, fear, and stress can affect your general health. For this reason, it's more advantageous to concentrate your efforts on what you can do to safeguard your pregnancy, such as maintaining your composure and relaxation, eating a healthy diet, and drinking enough water.

When you're ready to try again, embrace healthy pregnancy practices such as:

- **Taking care of any underlying health issues**. Do a thorough preconception examination if you haven't already. Untreated health issues like diabetes, hypertension, thyroid issues, and sexually transmitted infections might interfere with the pregnancy.

- **Manage your stress**. High levels of stress could make it more challenging to get pregnant. Find strategies to relax if you're feeling overly worried or anxious. Deep breathing, meditation, visualization, acupuncture, and yoga have positive effects.

- **Manage your alcohol and caffeine intake**. Avoid exceeding 200 mg of caffeine per day, as this may increase your chance of pregnancy loss. Stop drinking alcohol if you do. Alcohol may increase the likelihood of miscarriage and negatively impact fertility.

- **Quit smoking if you do.** Additionally, do your best to avoid third- or second-hand smoke.

Acknowledging your parental role in the deceased baby

If you choose to become pregnant again following pregnancy loss, please know that your unborn child is distinct from the baby who has passed away. You'll never forget your baby who died. You can still talk about the baby that was lost or call him or her by name. It has been shown that parents more readily free up emotional energy to accept a new baby by continuing to recognize their parenting role toward the infant who has passed away.

Talk to your unborn child about your pregnancy loss. A developing baby in the womb can recognize the mother's voice by term and hear at 16 weeks. The unborn child is aware of the world outside the womb. This can also make parents realize that their unborn child might feel their sorrow and their love and protection. This is such important bonding time. Talk to your unborn child about your pregnancy loss.

Nine

Conclusion

❤

Pregnancy loss is more common than the flu, but we still don't discuss it enough. There isn't a singular straight-forward explanation about why it happens, but one in six single or married women will miscarry at some point in their life. It cuts across cultures, social classes, different family dynamics, and religious beliefs. It may happen sooner or further along in the pregnancy. It has nothing to do with any-thing anyone did, so pregnancy loss shouldn't be as taboo as it seems.

Pregnancy loss is an actual loss, so it is sad when single women and couples experiencing this loss are left to grieve alone. In my opinion, nothing is more heartbreaking than needing the love, support, and comfort of loved ones and remaining a mother about it, while simultaneously being subjected to certain stereotypes and opinions. Making assumptions about anyone going through the painful tragedy of pregnancy loss is wrong, and we must do better as a society. We must all look beyond our fogged opinions about how people should mourn, act or grieve their losses and ask ourselves whether our views are justified or if they are nothing more than the result of ignorance and narrow-mindedness.

More women are going through miscarriages than many of us realize and understand; married, single, divorced, working through breakups, surrogates, celebrities (think Meghan Markle and Gabrielle Union), women in higher positions like CEOs and business owners, etc. And the reality of pregnancy loss and the subsequent grief is even worse in cultures where it is even more taboo to have sex before marriage.

The pain of pregnancy loss is unimaginable. Think about the feeling of coming into the hospital pregnant & leaving without a child, as is the case in stillbirth. This is just an experience I wouldn't wish on anyone. Why would we make such a conversation taboo? Why should we feel guilty for going through something so traumatic? Why should we let our loved ones grieve alone? We now know that women who've experienced pregnancy loss are more prone to depression, anxiety, PTSD, and other severe mental health disorders. Treating this sensitive topic as taboo is hurting us. What's the cost of silence and living your trauma through silence just to make people around you comfortable? Your mental health? Your happiness? The chance at healing and living your best life? Think about it.

If you or your loved one has lost a pregnancy, my heart breaks for you and wraps you in understanding, warmth, tenderness, and support. I pray, my dear friend, that you may find healing. You may never forget, but I hope the pain you feel as you read this may subside, over time, and not feel as intense as it is right now. I hope you find comfort and support in your loved ones and community. I hope you learn to accept, appreciate, and love yourself for who you are and feel comfortable in your skin. Grieve without restricting yourself to a specific timeline. Look for the beauty and blessing in your loss and heartbreak if you can. Indeed, "every cloud has a silver lining." I hope you find that.

I hope this book gives you the much-needed support and reminds you of how precious and beautiful you are as a woman. I sincerely hope you found reading it as enjoyable as I did creating it. If you did, please leave a genuine review on Amazon. This way, other women who've experienced this tragedy get to read it and benefit from its wisdom.

Until next time, my loves, stay hydrated, love yourself, and embrace your beauty.

Hugs and Love,

Heather Dolson, R.N.

Ten

References

Biali, S. (2022, July 1). *Creating Space for Grief and Loss | Psychology Today*. Psychology Today; www.psychologytoday.com. https://www.psychologytoday.com/us/blog/prescriptions-life/201606/creating-space-grief-and-loss

Chow, M. C. (2021, March 8). *15 Ways to Heal After A Miscarriage*. Birth Song Botanicals. Retrieved August 29, 2022, from https://www.birthsongbotanicals.com/blogs/birth-song-blog/heal-after-miscarriage

Newman, E. L. N. (2012, June). *Miscarriage and loss*. American Psychology Association. Retrieved August 29, 2022, from https://www.apa.org/monitor/2012/06/miscarriage

Dugas, Slane, C. D. V. H. S. (2022, June 27). *Miscarriage*. National Library of Medicine. Retrieved August 29, 2022, from https://www.ncbi.nlm.nih.gov/books/NBK532992/

Blomberg, C. B. [TED X Talks]. (2018, June 1). *Silently Suffering After Pregnancy Loss* [Video]. YouTube. https://www.yo utube.com/watch?v=l22udhFhsOE

CARDOZA, SCHNEIDER, K. C. A. R. D. O. Z. A. C. M. S. (2021, June 14). *The Importance Of Mourning Losses (Even When They Seem Small)*. Npr. Retrieved August 29, 2022, from https://www.npr.org/2021/06/02/1002446604/the-im portance-of-mourning-losses-even-when-they-seem-small

Gupta, S. G. (2022, April 16). *What Is Disenfranchised Grief?* VeryWell Mind. Retrieved August 29, 2022, from https://www.verywellmind.com/disenfranchised-grie f-definition-causes-impact-and-coping-5221901

Casabianca, S. S. C. (2021, February 11). *Mourning and the 5 Stages of Grief*. PsychCentral. Retrieved August 29, 2022, from https://psychcentral.com/lib/the-5-stages-of-loss-an d-grief#Going-through-the-5-stages-of-grief:-How-it-feels

World Health Organization. (n.d.). *Why we need to talk about losing a baby*. Retrieved August 29, 2022, from https://www.who.int/news-room/spotlight/why-we -need-to-talk-about-losing-a-baby

Benoist, K. B. (2021, January 21). *A Guide To Setting Boundaries*. I Don't Mind. Retrieved August 29, 2022, from https://idontmind.com/journal/a-guide-to-setting-boundaries

Gold, Sen, Hayward, K. G. A. S. R. H. (2010, April 5). *Marriage and Cohabitation Outcomes After Pregnancy Loss*. National Library of Medicine. Retrieved August 29, 2022, from https://www.ncbi.nlm.nih.gov/pmc/articles/PMC2883880/

Miller, Temple-Smith, Bilardi, E. J. M. M. J. T. J. E. B. (2019, May 5). *'There was just no-one there to acknowledge that it happened to me as well': A qualitative study of male partner's experience of miscarriage*. PLOS ONE. Retrieved August 29, 2022, from https://journals.plos.org/plosone/article?id=10.1371/journal.pone.0217395#sec024

March Of Dimes. (2017, October). *DEALING WITH GRIEF AFTER THE DEATH OF YOUR BABY*. March of Dimes. Retrieved August 29, 2022, from https://www.marchofdimes.org/complications/dealing-with-grief-after-the-death-of-your-baby.aspx

Collins, C., Riggs, D.W. & Due, C. (2014). The impact of pregnancy loss on women's adult relationships. Grief Matters: The Australian Journal of Grief and Bereavement, 17, 44-50.

Henderson, S. H. (2015, August 15). *Miscarriage as a single woman: No partner to cry with, but no marriage to keep afloat, either*. Washington Post. Retrieved August 29, 2022, from

https://www.washingtonpost.com/news/soloish/wp/2015/08/17/miscarriage-as-a-single-woman-no-partner-to-cry-with-but-no-marriage-to-keep-afloat-either/

Single Mothers by Choice. (n.d.). *Welcome to Single Mothers by Choice!®*. Retrieved August 29, 2022, from https://www.singlemothersbychoice.org/

Taylor, M. T. (2022, June 24). *Postpartum Recovery After a Pregnancy Loss*. What to Expect. Retrieved August 29, 2022, from

https://www.whattoexpect.com/pregnancy/pregnancy-loss/postpartum-recovery-symptoms-after-miscarriage/#:~:text=After%20a%20miscarriage%20or%20early,to%20give%20it%20another%20try

Bhardwaj, N. B. (2020, April 28). *7 things you must do after a miscarriage according to a gynaecologist*. Health Shots. Retrieved August 29, 2022, from

https://www.healthshots.com/preventive-care/reproductive-care/7-things-you-must-do-after-a-miscarriage-according-to-a-gynaecologist/

Taylor, M. T. (2022, January 28). *What Happens After a Still-birth and How to Cope*. What to Expect. Retrieved August 29, 2022, from https://www.whattoexpect.com/pregnancy/pregnancy-loss/stillbirth-recovery

Taylor, M. T. (2022, June 24). *What Happens After a Medical Termination of Pregnancy and How to Cope*. What to Expect. Retrieved August 29, 2022, from https://www.whattoexpect.com/pregnancy/pregnancy-loss/coping-after-a-medical-termination-of-pregnancy

Huberty, Leiferman, Gold, Rowedder, Cacciatore, McClain, J. H. J. A. L. K. J. G. L. R. J. C. D. B. M. (2014, November 29). *Physical activity and depressive symptoms after stillbirth: informing future interventions*. BMC Pregnancy and Childbirth. Retrieved August 29, 2022, from https://bmcpregnancychildbirth.biomedcentral.com/articles/10.1186/s12884-014-0391-1

Kharbanda, N. K. (2021, June 28). *Diet After Miscarriage: What To Eat And What Not For Healing*. Only My Health. Retrieved August 29, 2022, from https://www.onlymyhealth.com/diet-after-miscarriage-what-to-eat-and-what-to-avoid-1624882909

Chow, M. C. (201–03-08). *15 Ways to Heal After A Miscar-riage*. Birth Song Botanicals Co. Retrieved August 29, 2022, from https://www.birthsongbotanicals.com/blogs/birth-song-blog/heal-after-miscarriage

Côté -Arsenault D. & O'Leary, J. (2015). Understanding the experience of pregnancy subsequent to Perinatal loss. In: Wright, P, Limbo, R., Black, P (Eds.) Perinatal and Pediatric...

Gold, Leon, Boggs, Sen, K. J. G. I. L. M. E. B. A. S. (2016, March 1). *Depression and Posttraumatic Stress Symptoms After Peri-natal Loss in a Population-Based Sample*. National Library of Medicine. Retrieved August 29, 2022, from https://www.ncbi.nlm.nih.gov/pmc/articles/PMC4955602/

Brock, D. (2017, August 27). *When Dreams Die... Grieving What Should Have Been | The Grit and Grace Project*. The Grit and Grace Project; thegritandgraceproject.org. https://thegritandgraceproject.org/faith/grieving-what-should-have-been

Clarke, J. (n.d.). *5 stages of grief - Search*. 5 Stages of Grief - Search; www.bing.com. Retrieved August 26, 2022, from https://www.bing.com/search?q=5+stages+of+grief&qs=MT&pq=5+stages&sc=10-8&cvid=8BFB50A3540C41A4A3BD926CECEB5C42&FORM=QBRE&sp=1

CNN, M. V. (2021, July 15). *Miscarriage and men: Changing how we talk about loss - CNN*. CNN; edition.cnn.com. https://edition.cnn.com/2021/07/15/health/miscarriage-men-grief-loss-wellness/index.html

Dealing with Anger and Frustration | Mental Health America. (n.d.). Mental Health America; mhanational.org. Retrieved August 26, 2022, from https://mhanational.org/dealing-anger-and-frustration

Dealing With Anger in a Healthy Way Is Crucial. (2021, February 27). Verywell Mind; www.verywellmind.com . https://www.verywellmind.com/dos-and-donts-of-dealing-with-anger-3145081

Experiencing a pregnancy loss | Pregnancy Birth and Baby. (n.d.). Experiencing a Pregnancy Loss | Pregnancy Birth and Baby; www.pregnancybirthbaby.org.au. Retrieved August 26, 2022, from https://www.pregnancybirthbaby.org.au/experiencing-a-pregnancy-loss

For Men Dealing with Loss - Pregnancy & Infant Loss and Infertility Support. (n.d.). For Men Dealing with Loss - Pregnancy & Infant Loss and Infertility Support; longisland pregnancyandinfantloss.com. Retrieved August 26, 2022,

from https://longislandpregnancyandinfantloss.com/griev
ing-and-parenting-after-loss/for-men/

Grieving the Loss of Dreams. (n.d.). Grieving the Loss of
Dreams; theaquilareport.com. Retrieved August 26, 2022,
from https://theaquilareport.com/grieving-loss-dreams/

Grieving the Loss of Hopes and Dreams - Whats your Grief.
(2015, June 9). Whats Your Grief; whatsyourgrief.com. https
://whatsyourgrief.com/loss-of-hopes-and-dreams/

Hamby, S. (2022, July 1). Making Space for Grieving | Psychol-
ogy Today. Psychology Today; www.psychologytoday.com
. https://www.psychologytoday.com/us/blog/the-web-viol
ence/201501/making-space-grieving

How to Cope with Miscarriage. (n.d.). Healthline; www.heal
thline.com. Retrieved August 26, 2022, from https://www.h
ealthline.com/health/coping-with-miscarriage

How to Honor an Angel Baby After a Miscarriage — 11 Ways to
Honor a Lost Pregnancy. (n.d.). What to Expect;
www.whattoexpect.com. Retrieved August 26, 2022, from
https://www.whattoexpect.com/pregnancy/pregnancy-loss
/how-to-honor-lost-pregnancies/#:~:text=For%20some%20
women%2C%20finding%20a%20way%20to%20honor,jew

elry%20or%20plan%20a%20ceremony%20with%20close%20family.

Meaningful Grieving After Pregnancy Loss. (2013, June 10). Whats Your Grief; whatsyourgrief.com. https://whatsyourgrief.com/grieving-after-pregnancy-loss/

Men and miscarriage: Navigating grief after a pregnancy loss. (n.d.). Healthy Male; www.healthymale.org.au. Retrieved August 26, 2022, from https://www.healthymale.org.au/news/men-partner-miscarriage-guide-to-coping

Men on pregnancy and infant loss: Anger, crying in private and being expected to 'man up' - CNA Lifestyle. (n.d.). CNA Lifestyle; cnalifestyle.channelnewsasia.com. Retrieved August 26, 2022, from https://cnalifestyle.channelnewsasia.com/singapore/men-pregnancy-loss-baby-death-coping-anger-sadness-274251

Petriglieri, G. (2020, December 21). *Make Space for Grief After a Year of Loss.* Harvard Business Review; hbr.org. https://hbr.org/2020/12/make-space-for-grief-after-a-year-of-loss

Pregnancy Loss: Coping and Recovering. (n.d.). eMedicineHealth; www.emedicinehealth.com. Retrieved August 26, 2022, from https://www.emedicinehealth.com/pregnancy_loss/article_em.htm

Pregnancy Loss: Processing the Pain of Miscarriage. (n.d.). Pregnancy Loss: Processing the Pain of Miscarriage; www.linkedin.com. Retrieved August 26, 2022, from https://www.linkedin.com/pulse/pregnancy-loss-processing-pain-miscarriage-

Remembering your baby after a miscarriage | Tommy's. (n.d.). Remembering Your Baby after a Miscarriage | Tommy's; www.tommys.org. Retrieved August 26, 2022, from https://www.tommys.org/baby-loss-support/miscarriage-information-and-support/support-after-miscarriage/remembering-your-baby-after-miscarriage

Watson, S. (n.d.). *How to cope with pregnancy loss | BabyCenter.* BabyCenter; www.babycenter.com. Retrieved August 26, 2022, from https://www.babycenter.com/pregnancy/your-life/coping-with-pregnancy-loss_4006#:~:text=Losing%20a%20baby%20during%20pregnancy%20is%20a%20difficult,sadness%2C%20and%20shock.%20Everyone%20processes%20pregnancy%20loss%20differently.

Cronkleton, E. (n.d.). *Yoga for Stress: Breath, Poses, and Meditation to Calm Anxiety.* Healthline; www.healthline.com. Retrieved August 26, 2022, from https://www.healthline.com/health/fitness/yoga-for-stress

How Yoga Can Help Reduce Stress. (2020, March 30). Verywell Mind; www.verywellmind.com. https://www.verywellmind.com/how-yoga-can-help-reduce-stress-3567211#:~:text=Yoga%20has%20long%20been%20known%20to%20be%20a,this%20ancient%20practice%20brings%20to%20their%20stressful%20lives.

yoga alternatives - Search. (n.d.). Yoga Alternatives - Search; www.bing.com. Retrieved August 26, 2022, from https://www.bing.com/search?q=yoga+alternatives&qs=n&form=QBRE&sp=-1&pq=yoga+alternativ&sc=9-15&sk=&cvid=D96B597DA2C1422DAE9865ECB82338A1&ghsh=0&ghacc=0&ghpl=

Yoga as an alternative and complementary approach for stress management: a systematic review - PubMed. (2014, January 1). PubMed; pubmed.ncbi.nlm.nih.gov. https://pubmed.ncbi.nlm.nih.gov/24647380/

6 Steps to Release Shame and Finally Cultivate Self-Worth | Christiane Northrup, M.D. (2016, October 31). 6 Steps to Release Shame and Finally Cultivate Self-Worth | Christiane Northrup, M.D.; www.drnorthrup.com. https://www.drnorthrup.com/self-worth-release-shame/

7 Ways to Help Overcome Grief after Pregnancy Loss. (n.d.). FertilitySmarts; www.fertilitysmarts.com. Retrieved August 26, 2022, from https://www.fertilitysmarts.com/7-ways-to -help-overcome-grief-after-pregnancy-loss/2/2262

A.A., S. H. (2019, June 8). *How to Practice Self-Forgiveness When You Are Too Hard on Yourself - Learning Mind.* Learning Mind; www.learning-mind.com. https://www.learning-mind.com/how-to-practice-self-forgi veness-hard-on-yourself/#:~:text=1%20An%20Inner%20dia logue%20on%20paper.%20When%20you,they%20can%20 be%20large%20or%20small%2C%20doesn%E2%80%99t% 20matter.

Bliss, S. (2013, September 23). *Pregnancy as a Rite of Passage - Guardian Liberty Voice.* Guardian Liberty Voice; guardianlv .com. https://guardianlv.com/2013/09/pregnancy-as-a-rite -of-passage/

Brady, K. (2019, September 25). *7 Tips For Practicing Self-For- giveness - Keir Brady Counseling Services.* Keir Brady Coun- seling Services; keirbradycounseling.com. https://keirbrad ycounseling.com/self-forgiveness/

Cherry, K. (2021, February 17). *How to Forgive Yourself*. Very-well Mind; www.verywellmind.com. https://www.verywell mind.com/how-to-forgive-yourself-4583819

efffects of shame - Search. (n.d.). Efffects of Shame - Search; www.bing.com. Retrieved August 26, 2022, from https://www.bing.com/search?q=+efffects+of+shame&qs=n &form=QBRE&sp=-1&pq=efffects+of+shame&sc=1-17&sk=& cvid=71FEC7794EBC43A3A7A4C0256707143A&ghsh=0&gha cc=0&ghpl=

Exploring Shame | Made of Millions Foundation. (n.d.) . Made of Millions Foundation; www.madeofmillions.com. Retrieved August 26, 2022, from https://www.madeofmillio ns.com/articles/exploring-shame

Healing From Pregnancy Loss. (n.d.). Totum Healing Guides; guides.totumhealing.com. Retrieved August 26, 2022, from https://guides.totumhealing.com/courses/heali ng-from-pregnancy-loss-free-guide

Healing through Miscarriage, Stillbirth and Infertility - Pregn ancyLossHealing.com. (2016, May 16). Pregnancy Loss Heal-ing; pregnancylosshealing.com. https://pregnancylossheal ing.com/

Honoring Your Baby After Loss — Benefit Bump. (2021, March 11). Benefit Bump; www.benefitbump.com. https://www.benefitbump.com/perinatal-loss-content/honoringbaby#:~:text=%20Honoring%20Your%20Baby%20Afte r%20Loss%20%201,Some%20families%20choose%20to%2 0donate%20to...%20More%20

Jyn@FaithfulMotherhood, & . (2018, November 2). *7 Powerful Ways to Honor Your Lost Baby - Faithful Motherhood.* Faithful Motherhood; www.faithfulmotherhood.com. https://www.faithfulmotherhood.com/honoring-lost-baby/

Kripke, K. (2011, December 15). *Having A Baby After Infant Loss: The Mix of Grief & Joy.* POSTPARTUM PROGRESS; postpartumprogress.com . https://postpartumprogress.com/having-a-baby-after-infant-loss-the-complicated-mix-of-grief-joy

Northrup, C. (n.d.). *5 Steps To Release Shame And Move Forward To Self-Love.* 5 Steps To Release Shame And Move Forward To Self-Love by Dr. Christiane Northrup - HealYourLife; www.healyourlife.com. Retrieved August 26, 2022, from https://www.healyourlife.com/5-steps-to-release-shame-and-move-forward-to-self-love

Pregnancy After Loss: Having A Baby After Multiple Miscar-riages. (2018, November 16). Mama Natural; www.maman atural.com. https://www.mamanatural.com/pregnancy-aft er-loss/

Pregnancy and Infant Loss: Honoring a Lost Baby - Memorial Memories. (2021, December 8). Memorial Memories; memo rial-memories.com. https://memorial-memories.com/preg nancy-and-infant-loss-honoring-a-lost-baby/

Pregnancy loss and anxiety and depression during subse-quent pregnancies: data from the C-ABC study - PubMed. (2013, January 1). PubMed; pubmed.ncbi.nlm.nih.gov. http s://pubmed.ncbi.nlm.nih.gov/23146315/

Shekinah. (2019, September 26). *Pregnancy as a "Rite of Passage" - Shekinah Leigh.* Shekinah Leigh; shekinahleigh.com.au. https://shekinahleigh.com.au/pregnancy-as-a-rite-of-passa ge/#:~:text=Pregnancy%20as%20a%20%E2%80%9CRite%2 0of%20Passage%E2%80%9D%20Originally%20posted,with %20the%20support%20of%20her%20family%20and%20c ommunity.

Taughinbaugh, C. (2014, August 4). *7 Ways to Release the Shame That is Holding You Back - Cathy Taughinbaugh |*

Treatment Talk. Cathy Taughinbaugh | Treatment Talk; c athytaughinbaugh.com. https://cathytaughinbaugh.com/7 -ways-to-release-the-shame-that-is-holding-you-back/

The Effects of Shame | 121hypnosis.com. (n.d.). The Effects of Shame | 121hypnosis.Com; www.121hypnosis.com. Retrieved August 26, 2022, from https://www.121hypnosis.com/the-effects-of-shame/#:~:te xt=%20The%20Effects%20of%20Shame%20%201%20Sha me,at%20the%20heart%20of%20shame.%20The...%20Mor e%20

Therapy and Pregnancy Loss - The Healing Collective. (2019, October 9). The Healing Collective; www.healingcollective .ca. https://www.healingcollective.ca/general/therapy-and -pregnancy-loss/

Trying to Get Pregnant Again After a Miscarriage. (2020, May 28). Verywell Family; www.verywellfamily.co m. https://www.verywellfamily.com/having-a-baby-after-a -miscarriage-2759665

Ways to honor a baby who dies in pregnancy or infancy |
BabyCenter. (n.d.). BabyCenter; www.babycenter.com. Retrieved August 26, 2022, from

https://www.babycenter.com/pregnancy/your-life/honorin
g-a-baby-who-dies-in-pregnancy-or-infancy_10339724

What Is Shame? (2021, May 27). Verywell Mind; www.verywe
llmind.com. https://www.verywellmind.com/what-is-sham
e-5115076

*Why Your Whole Self Feels Ashamed But Only Part of You Feels
Guilty.* (2021, February 18). Verywell Mind; www.verywellm
ind.com. https://www.verywellmind.com/what-is-shame-4
25328

When to Try for Another Baby After Stillbirth. (2021, May 13).
Verywell Family; www.verywellfamily.com.
https://www.verywellfamily.com/when-is-it-safe-to-conceiv
e-after-stillbirth-2371776#:~:text=Giving%20birth%20to%2
0another%20baby%20isn%27t%20a%20cure-all,decide%2
0to%20embark%20on%20another%20pregnancy%20or%2
0not.

Baby loss statistics | Tommy's. (n.d.). Baby Loss Statistics
| Tommy's; www.tommys.org. Retrieved August 26, 2022,
from https://www.tommys.org/baby-loss-support/pregna
ncy-loss-statistics

Brook, W. (2020, April 30). *Expressing Grief is a Personal
Process that Takes Time – Adria's Notebook.* Expressing Grief

Is a Personal Process That Takes Time – Adria's Notebook; b logs.iu.edu. https://blogs.iu.edu/adriasnotebook/2020/04/30/expressing-grief-is-a-personal-process-that-takes-time/

CDC. (2020, August 13). *Pregnancy and Infant Loss | CDC.* Centers for Disease Control and Prevention; www.cdc.gov . https://www.cdc.gov/ncbddd/stillbirth/features/pregnancy-infant-loss.html

Danielsson, K. (2020, January 21). *No Amount of Alcohol Is Safe During Pregnancy.* Verywell Family; www.verywellfamily.com. https://www.verywellfamily.com/alcohol-pregnancy-and-miscarriage-risks-2371444

Dealing With Hurtful Words - Proctor Gallagher Institute. (2021, April 30). Proctor Gallagher Institute; www.proctorgallagherinstitute.com. https://www.proctorgallagherinstitute.com/25392/dealing-with-hurtful-words

donny. (2015, August 18). *5 simple tips to deal with hurtful words.* 5 Simple Tips to Deal with Hurtful Words – HisVoiceOnline.Com; hisvoiceonline.com. https://hisvoiceonline.com/simple-steps-to-overcome-hurtful-words/

Eldridge, L. (2020, January 13). *The Dangers of Passive Smoking.* Verywell Health; www.verywellhealth.com. https://www.verywellhealth.com/information-about-passiv

e-smoking-2249146#:~:text=Passive%20smoking%20while
%20pregnant%20increases%20the%20risk%20of,to%20an
%20increased%20incidence%20of%20congenital%20heart
%20defects.

Gance, L. (n.d.). *Finding Support After Pregnancy Loss | The
Yinova Center*. Finding Support After Pregnancy Loss | The
Yinova Center; www.yinovacenter.com. Retrieved August 26,
2022, from https://www.yinovacenter.com/blog/finding-su
pport-and-healing-after-pregnancy-loss/

Harrison, K. (n.d.). *7 Ways to Help Overcome Grief after
Pregnancy Loss*. FertilitySmarts; www.fertilitysmarts.com.
Retrieved August 26, 2022, from
https://www.fertilitysmarts.com/7-ways-to-help-overcome
-grief-after-pregnancy-loss/2/2262#:~:text=%207%20Ways
%20to%20Help%20Overcome%20Grief%20after,It%20sou
nds%20so%20simple%2C%20and%20yet...%20More%20

Heflick, N. (2022, July 1). *Expressing Grief vs. Holding it in |
Psychology Today*. Psychology Today; www.psychologytod
ay.com. https://www.psychologytoday.com/us/blog/the-b
ig-questions/201305/expressing-grief-vs-holding-it-in

How to Cope With Hurtful Insults: 15 Steps (with Pictures). (2021, June 9). wikiHow; www.wikihow.com. https://www. wikihow.com/Cope-With-Hurtful-Insults

Launder, M. (2021, January 19). *Support after pregnancy loss: how you can help - Nursing in PracticeNursing in Practice.* Nursing in Practice; www.nursinginpractice.com . https://www.nursinginpractice.com/clinical/womens-hea lth/support-after-pregnancy-loss-how-you-can-help/

Life, N. (2020, October 16). *Expressing Grief | New Life.* New Life; newlife.com. https://newlife.com/expressing-grief/

Mclean-Green, K. (2015, September 4). *Can Alcohol Cause a Miscarriage?* Absolute Advocacy; www.absoluteadvocac y.org. https://www.absoluteadvocacy.org/can-alcohol-cau se-a-miscarriage/

Meaningful Grieving After Pregnancy Loss. (2013, June 10). Whats Your Grief; whatsyourgrief.com. https://whatsyourgr ief.com/grieving-after-pregnancy-loss/

Orgeron, T. (2019, January 8). *The Benefit of Support Groups. By: Terra Orgeron | by if me editors | if me | Medium.* Medium; medium.com. https://medium.com/ifme/the-benefit-of-support-groups-8 29fe0e77518#:~:text=Benefits%20of%20participating%20in

%20support%20groups%20may%20include%3A,to%20exp ect%20with%20your%20situation%20More%20items...%2 0

Pregnancy loss | Office on Women's Health. (2021, February 22). Pregnancy Loss | Office on Women's Health; www.wo menshealth.gov. https://www.womenshealth.gov/pregnan cy/youre-pregnant-now-what/pregnancy-loss

Rothschild, M. (2020, May 1). grief, grief awareness, grief recovery, grief coach, grief coach certification. GlobalGriefInstitute; www.globalgriefinstitute.com. https://www.globalgriefinstitute.com/post/expressing-grief -what-to-know-and-how-to-help-men-women-and-childre n-cope-with-grief

Scaccia, A. (n.d.). Pregnant and Alone: Tips for Support. Healthline; www.healthline.com. Retrieved August 26, 2022, from https://www.healthline.com/health/pregnancy/preg nant-and-alone-tips

Shaffstall, D. (2017, February 28). 5 Benefits of Grief and Bereavement Support Groups. 5 Benefits of Grief and Bereavement Support Groups; www.generationshcm.com . https://www.generationshcm.com/blog/2017/02/5-benef its-grief-bereavement-support-groups

Statistics – Facts about Miscarriage. (2007, September 19). Statistics – Facts about Miscarriage; pregnancyloss.info. htt ps://pregnancyloss.info/statistics/

Support groups helping women through pregnancies after loss - PubMed. (2004, October 1). PubMed; pubmed.ncbi.n lm.nih.gov. https://pubmed.ncbi.nlm.nih.gov/15359076/

The Advantages of Support Groups and Why You Should Join One - Kentucky Counseling Center. (2021, October 22). Kentucky Counseling Center; kentuckycounselingcenter.co m. https://kentuckycounselingcenter.com/advantages-of-s upport-groups-and-why-you-should-join-one/

Support Groups: Types, Benefits, and What to Expect - HelpG uide.org. (2021, October 1). HelpGuide.Org; www.helpguide .org. https://www.helpguide.org/articles/therapy-medicati on/support-groups.htm

Susman, D. (2015, April 23). *9 Benefits of Support Groups | Advocating for Better Mental Health.* Advocating for Bet- ter Mental Health | David Susman, PhD; davidsusman.com . https://davidsusman.com/2015/04/23/9-benefits-of-supp ort-groups/

Swindoll, C. (2020, April 26). *Expressing Grief*. Expressing
Grief; www.insight.org. https://www.insight.org/resources/
daily-devotional/individual/expressing-grief1

Vasquez, JD, CT, Dr. A. (2021, July 2). *10 Common Ways to
Express Grief in Public or Private | Cake Blog*. 10 Common
Ways to Express Grief in Public or Private | Cake Blog;
www.joincake.com.
https://www.joincake.com/blog/expressing-grief/#:~:text=
%20Different%20Ways%20You%20Can%20Publicly%20Exp
ress%20Grief,grief%20openly%20and%20publicly%20is%2
0to...%20More%20

Villines, Z. (n.d.). *Miscarriage rates by week*. Miscarriage
Rates by Week: Risks and Statistics;
www.medicalnewstoday.com. Retrieved August 26, 2022,
from
https://www.medicalnewstoday.com/articles/322634#:~:te
xt=The%20average%20risk%20of%20miscarriage%20by%
20the%20age,About%20a%2050%20percent%20chance%2
0of%20pregnancy%20loss

Davis, J. L. (n.d.). Couples May Change After Miscarriage. Retrieved August 29, 2022, from WebMD website: https://www.webmd.com/baby/news/20031008/coup
les-may-change-after-miscarriage

Board |, the B. M. A. (n.d.). Gentle exercise after pregnancy loss. Retrieved August 29, 2022, from BabyCentre UK website: https://www.babycentre.co.uk/a1014806/gentle-exercise-after-pregnancy-loss#:~:text=Exercise%20may%20be%20the%20last

Also By Heather Dolson

I created a companion guide to further support you on your path to wholeness and provide tangible tools so you can access your own inner wisdom and healer.

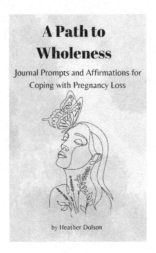

What you can expect in the guide:

- Tips for loving and deep self-care and ways to make time and space for journal practice.

- Journal prompts that guide you to look within yourself and do the soul work to process the heavy emotions and get it out of you in a black and white way.

- Affirmations that uplift and inspire you to love and accept yourself the way you are and give you hope for the future.

- Inclusive language for attached or single women and all situations.

- A rich resource that you can turn to in times of distress, sadness, isolation and feel held and loved.

If you are already saying "I don't stick to journaling," this book is broken down into sections and makes it easy to digest and attainable, even for 5 minutes a day.

Feeling whole after loss is possible. You are your best teacher, healer, and guide and this is the tool that can support you anytime, anywhere.

Find the companion guide on Amazon to buy.

I work with clients holistically to release trauma, quiet their minds, and listen to their intuition to step into their own creative power in life. I offer some free resources on my website.

- A 5-part *Quiet Your Mind* mini-video series www.hea theronhealth.com/quiet-your-mind

- A 1-hour training, *How to Find Peace Even When Sh*t Hits the Fan* www.heatheronhealth.com/free

- A 30-minute introduction to yoga and cannabis, *Radiant Conscious Cannabis Masterclass* www.heathe ronhealth.com/cannabismasterclass

Feel free to take advantage of any of these free resources to ease anxious thoughts, relieve emotional overwhelm, and finally give yourself the deep, loving self-care you have been craving.

Printed in Great Britain
by Amazon